Hip Disorders
in Children

POSTGRADUATE ORTHOPAEDICS SERIES

under the General Editorship of

A. Graham Apley, MB, BS, FRCS

Honorary Director, Department of Orthopaedics, St. Thomas' Hospital, London; Consultant Orthopaedic Surgeon, The Rowley Bristow Orthopaedic Hospital, Pyrford and St. Peter's Hospital, Chertsey, Surrey

Hip Disorders
in Children

G.C. LLOYD-ROBERTS

MChir(Cantab), FRCS(England)
Orthopaedic Surgeon, The Hospital for Sick Children,
Great Ormond Street, London

A.H.C. RATLIFF

ChM(Bristol), FRCS(England)
Consultant Orthopaedic Surgeon, United Bristol Hospitals

Butterworths
LONDON-BOSTON
Sydney-Wellington-Durban-Toronto

First Published 1978
Reprinted 1981

British Library Cataloguing in Publication Data

Lloyd – Roberts, George Charles
    Hip disorders in children – (Postgraduate
    orthopaedics series).
    1. Hip joint – Diseases
    2. Children – Diseases
    I. Title   II. Series   III. Ratliff, A H C
    617'.58   RJ480   77–30339

    ISBN 0 407 00132 8

Typeset by Butterworths Litho Preparation Department
Printed in Great Britain by Hartnoll Print Ltd., Bodmin, Cornwall

Editor's Foreword

The traditional tome is ill-suited to dealing with those aspects of orthopaedics which are controversial and advancing rapidly. However massive the manual, the space available for detailed appraisal of individual topics can never be enough. The *Postgraduate Orthopaedics Series* aims to cover such topics in individual books – monographs of modest size, published as and when the need becomes apparent. For each subject one or two authorities are invited to survey the recent literature and to use it as a backcloth against which to present their own views, based on personal observations and technical know-how.

In this, the first volume of the series, two writers of distinction and experience have combined to describe disorders of the growing hip; each has extensive knowledge in this important field and they have included an up-to-the-minute account of their practice and results. Their constant collaboration was of course encouraged and fostered, but each was asked to write his particular sections single-handed, so that the individual flavour is retained. I enjoyed both and have learned much from them.

A. G. A.

Acknowledgements

The authors are indebted to the Departments of Medical Illustration of Bristol Royal Infirmary and the Hospital for Sick Children, London. They also thank their secretaries Mrs S. McLennan, Mrs C. Calder, Mrs B. Warren and Mrs S. Miers for their invaluable assistance in the preparation of this work.

Publishers' note

Owing to the age of some of the x-ray originals and the fact that the subjects are children, the reproduction of certain of the illustrations is unavoidably imperfect. The position of the right and left hips has been reversed in a few of the illustrations. However, the 'message' they convey is in no instance ambiguous.

Contents

1

Congenital Femoral Deficiency

G. C. Lloyd- Roberts

Femoral dysplasia is a maldevelopment of broad spectrum, including not only deficiencies of the femur ranging from minor shortening to total absence, but also modifications in form such as coxa vara, pseudarthrosis and hip dislocation. Furthermore the dysplasia may not be restricted to the femur alone but be a reflection of a generalized malformation of the whole limb so that abnormalities of the leg and foot complicate the problems of management. Lastly, the presentation may be bilateral with differing patterns of deformity on the two sides.

In so complex a disorder accurate classification of the numerous variations is essential, for the prognosis differs between one pattern and another. Denied this knowledge we cannot plan our management in a rational manner.

Prostheses will be an essential adjuvant in most cases but in this chapter I will consider only the role of surgery in preventing some predictable complications which will emerge as growth proceeds and in alleviating their effects later, in the hope that the problems facing the prosthetist will thereby be reduced.

Aetiology

A precise cause is not recognized and there is no genetic formula, but it seems that some noxious physical, chemical or infective influence may modify normal development at a vulnerable stage at some time before the ninth week of uterine life when the hip joint and femur become fully differentiated. The sequence of normal development has been well described and illustrated by King (1969).

Femoral dysplasia has been described following thalidomide poisoning (Fixsen and Lloyd-Roberts, 1974) and as one of the syndromes associated with maternal diabetes (Kucera, Lenz and Maier, 1965). It is therefore interesting to note that femoral deficiency has followed insulin injections into the yolk sac of developing chick embryos on the sixth day (Duraiswami, 1952). Morgan and Somerville (1960) have proposed an alternative explanation for the more proximal deficiencies postulating that the orderly progression of vascular invasion is arrested late in foetal life so that ossification in the cartilaginous model is delayed and the capacity for longitudinal growth greatly impaired.

1

Clinical features at birth

These vary with the degree of malformation. Those destined to develop simple femoral shortening alone will show no abnormality, whereas those in whom the hip joint and the greater part of the femur are absent will seem to have no femur and lack stability between the lower leg and pelvis. Most, however, display marked femoral shortening with flexion, abduction and external rotation deformity at the hip which is however stable and mobile from the position of fixed deformity — *Figure 1.1* — findings which may cause surprise when the radiograph

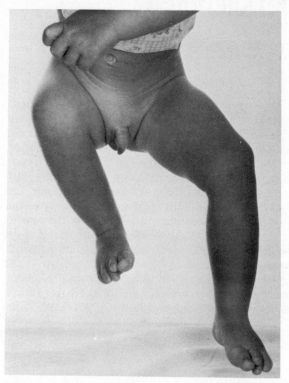

Figure 1.1. The leg is short, flexed, abducted and externally
rotated

is seen. These features are important for they indicate that continuity exists between femur and pelvis in spite of radiological translucency in the area normally occupied by the proximal femoral shaft (*Figure 1.2*).

Associated abnormalities when present may be local or general. Tibial shortening with fibular dysplasia is more likely to be seen in company with either severe femoral deficiency or in association with simple short femur when it takes precedence and dominates the clinical problem (Hootnick, *et al.*, 1976).

It would be surprising if an insult to the embryo during the stage of differentiation was localized in its effect and we must therefore be alert to the possibility of developmental anomalies elsewhere, especially in the arms.

Difficulty in diagnosis is unlikely when the manifestation is florid but in minor degrees, i.e. simple short femur and coxa vara, this is possible. A healed birth fracture will not show evidence of distal femoral epiphyseal delay and the shortening, if any, will not progress. Idiopathic hemiatrophy will declare itself

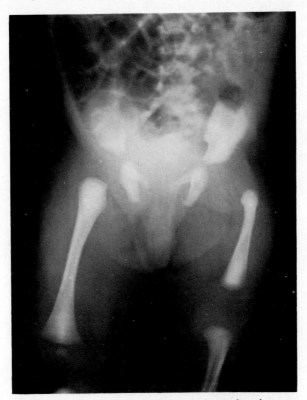

Figure 1.2. The proximal femur is translucent but the acet-abulum is well formed. The femur has not moved proximally and its tip is bulbous being situated at a greater distance from the acetabulum than on the normal side

in later childhood and is not identifiable in infancy, but the shortening and loss of girth characteristic of spinal dysraphism may be confusing as may unexplained dystrophy of a limb without the stigmata of femoral dysplasia. Congenital coxa vara must be distinguished from the infantile variety (*see below*).

CLASSIFICATION OF FEMORAL DYSPLASIA WITH SPECIAL REFERENCE TO THE PROGNOSIS OF THE HIP

It has already been emphasized that classification is essential to prognosis and prognosis is the key to management. Important contributions to the differentiation of types have been made by Aitken (1969) and Amstutz (1969) with others in a Symposium devoted to this subject which is probably the most significant publication on femoral dysplasia at the present time. Simple short femur and congenital coxa vara have been separately studied by Ring (1959, 1961) and Amstutz and Wilson (1962). The following observations are largely based upon the contributions of these authors.

Aitken's classification distinguishes four subdivisions of established deformity of increasing severity with instability (A–D) (*Figure 1.3*). Amstutz provides

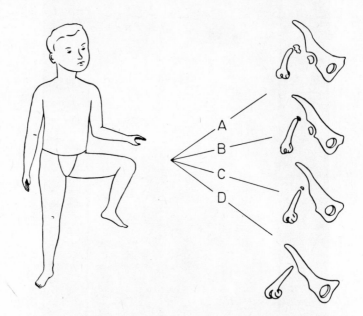

Figure 1.3. Aitken classification. (Reproduced with permission from *Proximal Femoral Focal Deficiency: A Congenital Anomaly.* 1969. Washington: National Academy of Sciences)

this in more detailed form, also arranged in terms of progressively severe dysplasia, as Types I–V with subdivisions illustrating the initial state and the final outcome in all, with alternatives in two of the Types described (*Figure 1.4*). Although more complex, the Amstutz classification is more apposite to the practical problems of management especially as applied to the hip and will therefore be adopted in the following discussion. Congenital short femur (simple hypoplasia) will be mentioned separately.

I will also incorporate certain observations which we have made with special reference to the signs by which those destined to develop pelvifemoral instability may be detected at a very early age (Fixsen and Lloyd-Roberts, 1974).

I intend, however, to make a further modification because this chapter deals primarily with surgical management of the hip which will, in the early stages, be concentrated upon the maintenance or restoration of stability with mobility within this joint. Consequently I will consider the various Types in relation to their influence upon the integrity of the hip joint, with special reference to the

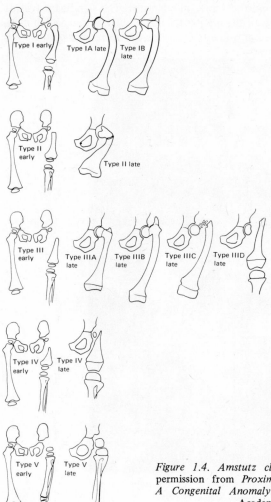

Figure 1.4. Amstutz classification. (Reproduced with permission from *Proximal Femoral Focal Deficiency: A Congenital Anomaly.* 1969. Washington: National Academy of Sciences)

indications for operations designed to preserve or restore this integrity. We may classify the indications for such operations in relation to the type of dysplasia as:

(a) Impossible;
(b) Indicated early;
(c) Indicated later;
(d) Unnecessary.

(a) *Hip joint reconstruction impossible (Amstutz Type V)*

The femur may very rarely be completely absent (Ring, 1961) but usually, although apparently absent at birth, later ossification will disclose persistence of the distal femoral epiphysis and the supracondylar area. The significant feature is absence of both components of the hip joint, i.e. femoral head and acetabulum. This can usually be recognized at an early stage for the acetabular concavity is

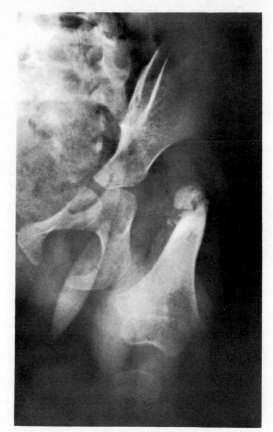

Figure 1.5. The acetabulum is flat indicating that the femoral head is absent

non-existent or greatly reduced implying lack of the femoral head. The knee joint, however is normal. The prospect for establishing a stable and mobile hip is clearly non-existent (*Figures 1.5 and 1.19*).

(b) *Hip joint reconstruction indicated early (Amstutz Type IV)*

The femur is at first represented by opacity limited to the distal third but it will ossify proximally with time. A concave acetabulum is present and the capital epiphysis will appear later. The appearance and position of the most proximal area of ossified femur is of importance. When this is pointed or irregular with sclerosis of the femur immediately distal to it, disintegration of the junction between bone and the cartilage model of the hip is imminent (*Figure 1.6*).

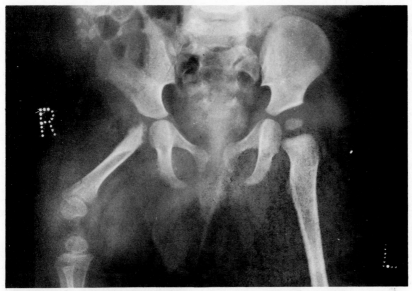

Figure 1.6. (a) The acetabulum is present. The proximal femur is pointed, sclerotic and closely opposed to the pelvis, cf. Figure 1.2.

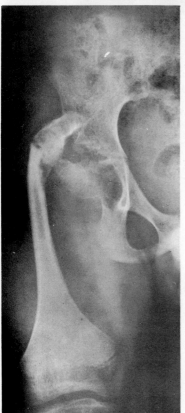

Figure 1.6. (b) The probable outcome if untreated. Note the well formed head in the acetabulum

Sometimes the femoral shaft is separated by a translucent line from a mushroom-like tuft proximally. This line represents the site of pseudarthrosis and the area of impending displacement (*Figure 1.7*) (Fixsen and Lloyd-Roberts, 1974). When weight is taken displacement occurs and the femur moves proximally and

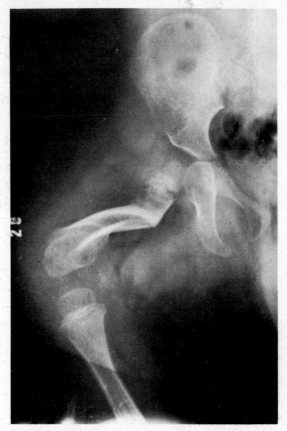

Figure 1.7. The proximal femur was tufted distal to the line of pseudarthrosis which can now be seen

inwards towards the pelvis. Operation is therefore indicated before walking begins (*Figure 1.8*). A further unusual indication was presented by a patient with an intact but very short femur in firm continuity with the capital epiphysis in whom the hip was found to be dislocated (*Figure 1.16*).

(c) *Hip joint reconstruction indicated later (Amstutz Types III BCD, II later and IB late)*

　　(1) Subtrochanteric pseudarthrosis is seen in the presence of an intact hip joint proximally and a short but intact femur distally. Some will heal

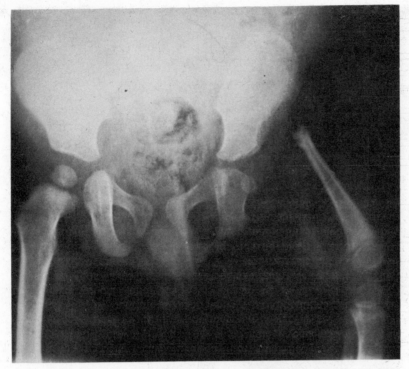

Figure 1.8. Displacement has taken place at the pseudarthrosis on walking. Note the head in the acetabulum

spontaneously but others persist so that coxa vara arising from sub-trochanteric angulation develops. Operation is indicated if any displacement is seen (*Figure 1.9*).

(2) Congenital coxa vara. This is the most complex group and the most difficult to categorize because of the variability and delay in presentation, uncertain outlook and confusion with the infantile (developmental) variety.

There are two broad patterns of congenital coxa vara. First we may encounter a situation less aggressive than that found in Type IV in which, as already noted, disintegration is early and rapid and occurs before the cervical and trochanteric areas are visible. In contrast we now see a coxa vara with either apparently satisfactory development of continuity between hip and femoral shaft or separated by an area of persistent translucency resembling a wide epiphyseal plate. In the first instance the femoral neck may gradually attenuate, bending into varus until ultimately contact is lost. In the second, although displacement occurs continuity is maintained. The area of translucency represents a persistent though relatively stable pseudarthrosis which finally heals (*Figure 1.10*).

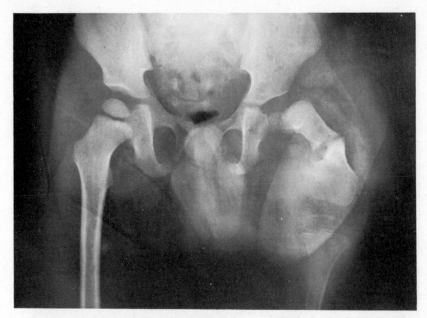

*Figure 1.9. (a) Subtrochanteric
pseudarthrosis with displacement*

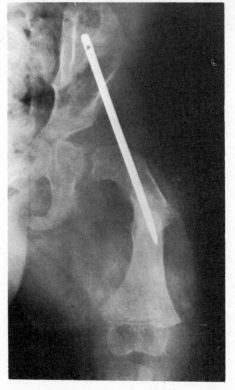

*Figure 1.9. (b) Union following nailing
and grafting. The nail has migrated
during healing. (Left side)*

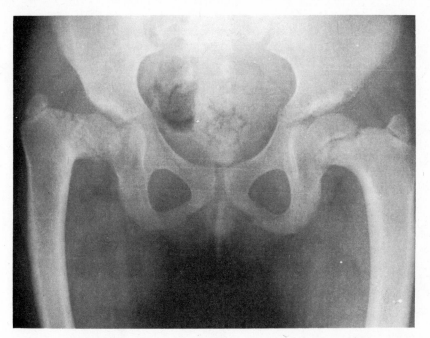

Figure 1.10. Coxa vara with a relatively stable healing defect in the neck

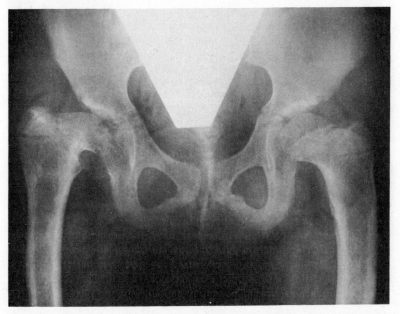

Figure 1.11. Coxa vara. On the right there is a deficient acetabulum with malformation and subluxation of the femoral head.

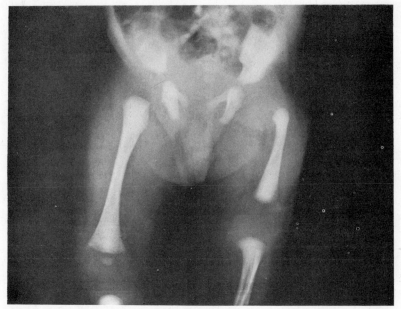

(a) (i)

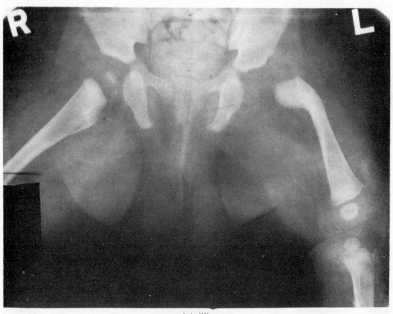

(a) (ii)

Figure 1.12. (a) Femoral deficiency of good prognosis in infancy (i) and at six months (ii)

12

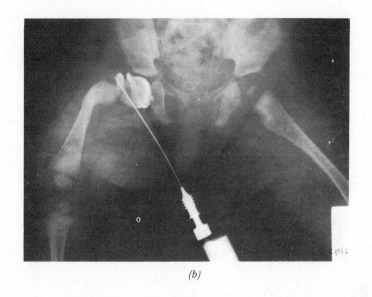

(b)

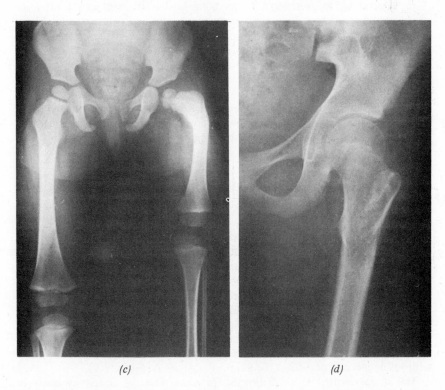

(c)   *(d)*

*Figure 1.12. (b) The arthrogram outlines the femoral head. (c) The outcome without treat-
ment, early and (d) late*

This second pattern of displacement in continuity may complicate simple femoral hypoplasia for which operation is not otherwise necessary (*see below*). The femoral head is at first spherical with a neck-shaft angle of around 90° which has all the appearances of stability. Lateral bowing of the femur, however, causes a relative increase in varus in the erect position. The head contour changes insidiously and becomes bullet-like; equally insidiously the acetabulum fails to develop, the head subluxates and the appearances closely resemble congenital subluxation with femoral head deformity. The acetabular failure may be a component of the syndrome as a whole or it may be due to abnormal pressure upon the developing socket imposed by deformity of the femoral head – a situation analogous to that seen in some patients with Perthes' disease with flattened and extruding heads. I suspect that it is a combination of the two (*Figure 1.11*).

The relationship between infantile coxa vara and the congenital type described above is difficult to assess. The subluxating and attenuating varieties are in no way comparable but there are certain similarities between them when mild deformity without acetabular deficiency follows persistence of relatively stable cervical pseudarthroses. The complications, such as subluxation, total displacement and extreme shortening characteristic of the congenital but absent in the infantile may be no more than a property of the degree of dysplasia (Golding, 1948). Blockey (1969) has discussed this dilemma emphasizing the differences and submitting convincing evidence that all the characteristics of the infantile type may be seen in patients who have had injuries to this area in infancy. The problem of aetiology remains unresolved but the clinical features are so widely divergent that it is better for practical purposes to distinguish between the congenital and infantile types of coxa vara. Both varieties, however, may require surgical treatment at some stage in their developmental progress.

(d) *Hip joint reconstruction unnecessary (Amstutz Types IA late and some Type II)*

The radiological features which distinguish proximal deficiency with a good prognosis, i.e. progressive ossification of the cartilaginous model resulting in stability and mobility of the hip without significant deformity, are again recognizable at a very early stage. The visible proximal stump of the femur is rounded and bulbous without spike, tuft or irregularity. It is opposite or just below the level of the acetabulum and separated from it by a translucent interval greater than that on the other side to accommodate the unossified cartilage model of the hip. Sclerosis is central in the shaft which may be angulated at this point (*Figures 1.12* and *1.2*). Surgical intervention is not necessary unless pseudarthrosis occurs and persists at the point of angulation (*Figure 1.9*).

The characteristics which distinguish proximal femoral deficiency likely to remain stable from those expected to displace are summarized below (Fixsen and Lloyd-Roberts, 1974) (*Figure 1.13*).

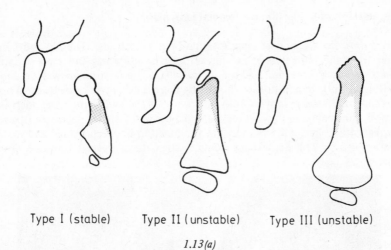

Type I (stable)   Type II (unstable)   Type III (unstable)

1.13(a)

Type	Appearance	Number of hips	Stable	Unstable
I	Bulbous	12	12	0
II	Tuft or cap	13	3	10
III	Not bulbous, no cap	5	0	5

1.13(b)

	Number of hips	Stable	Unstable
Distance greater than the normal side	15	10	5
Distance equal to the normal side	2	0	2
Distance less than the normal side	3	1	2

1.13(c)

Figure 1.13. (a) Line drawings of stable and unstable types. The shaded area represents the site of sclerosis. (b) The appearance of the proximal femur related to prognosis. (c) The distance between proximal femur and acetabulum related to prognosis. (Reproduced from Fixsen and Lloyd-Roberts, *J. Bone Jt Surg.* **56B** with permission)

Congenital short femur (Simple femoral hypoplasia)

This represents the mildest manifestation of the syndrome. The hip and femur differ from the normal only insofar as there is shortening and some variation from the normal bone architecture of the shaft. The features are well described by Ring (1959). In addition to shortening there is a delay in ossification at both proximal and distal epiphyses with narrowing of the medullary canal, increased cortical thickening and sometimes lateral bowing of trivial degree (c.f. severe bowing with congenital coxa vara) at the junction of the proximal and middle thirds (*Figure 1.14*). Some have no such stigmata of dysplasia but are simply short.

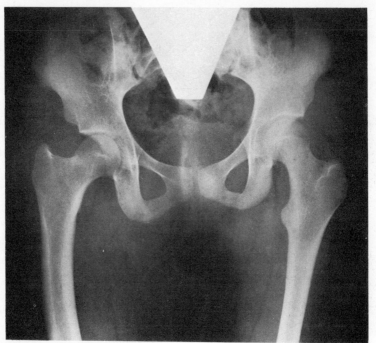

Figure 1.14. Congenital short femur with sure coxa vara compared with the normal. Note the lateral bowing and cortical sclerosis in the shaft

The prognosis is good apart from shortening which seldom exceeds 2 inches (5 cm). The discrepancy is consistent throughout growth so that the ultimate inequality of leg length may be predicted with accuracy by relating the proportionate shortening in childhood to the length of the appropriate parent's femur.

Two features which may escape early recognition modify the prognosis profoundly. Firstly, we must exclude an associated coxa vara which will immediately alter the classification to Type I or III (Amstutz) with implications of severe shortening and possibly progressive coxa vara or hip subluxation. Secondly a simple femoral shortening is commonly associated with congenital shortening of the tibia which may increase the final discrepancy by 4 to 5 inches. (10–13 cm) (Hootnick *et al.*, 1977).

Miscellaneous observations

It may be helpful to quantify the expected length discrepancy in the different varieties. It has already been observed that this seldom exceeds 2 in (~5.1 cm) in simple shortening, but if there is true femoral dysplasia with coxa vara we may anticipate 4 in (~10.2 cm). If this is complicated by pseudarthrosis we may add 2 in (~5.1 cm) to give a 6-in (~15.2 cm) discrepancy. The most severe (Amstutz IV and V) will be between 8 and 12 in (~20 and 30 cm) short.

The relative incidence of the patterns already described is difficult to assess and varies between published series. In general terms, however, the incidence is in inverse proportion to the severity. Thus simple femoral shortening is seen most frequently and total absence is very rare as is dislocation of an intact but deficient femur. Stable coxa vara predominates over the delayed onset unstable type.

Bilateral involvement is not uncommon and fortunately tends to be symmetrical, spanning the spectrum from bilateral simple shortening to total or subtotal deficiency. In some, however, the malformations are asymmetrical with inequality of leg length.

The morphological patterns described above will enable most to be categorized within one type or another. It is not in the nature of matters biological to permit rigid classification without divergence and thus from time to time we encounter a pattern which is not readily identifiable. On these occasions we can do no more than advise, somewhat lamely, that the condition be treated on its merits.

TECHNICAL CONSIDERATIONS IN SURGICAL TREATMENT

Having described the broad principles upon which we base our indications for operation to preserve hip joint function we must now consider extending operative indications to alleviate some other components of femoral deficiency and amplify some of the recommendations already proposed.

Although we are generally unable to influence the shortening effectively we can and should attempt when possible to alleviate the final handicap by concentrating upon prevention of instability in those predestined to this complication, or restoring stability when this is already lost. We now have useful classifications of the ultimate abnormalities in untreated patients and some knowledge of those signs which help us to predict in the very young the final outcome.

Having established the indications for early surgical treatment we must consider the surgical techniques available in the early stages to prevent undesirable developments from occurring during growth and also those designed to reduce the disability when deformity is established in older children. These operations should not be assessed in isolation but in relation to the remarkable developments in prosthetic science in recent years. Some form of prosthesis will be necessary in all but a few of those with simple femoral shortening, for the discrepancy is otherwise beyond surgical redemption. It is essential therefore that surgical and prosthetic aids be regarded as complementary rather than exclusive.

General principles of surgical treatment

Management is dominated by our ability to predict the outcome in the type of dysplasia with which we are dealing. Surgical and prosthetic modes are used concurrently and are at all times complementary. The surgeon should restrain his enthusiasm to undertake a challenging operation until the prosthetist has assured him that the success of the proposed procedure will in no way compromise his future programme. Surgical failure will usually be harmless, for the situation will revert to its original state, but partial success may, for example, result in a stable but stiff hip with deformity, whereas before there was mobility, albeit with instability. The surgeon must weigh the issues carefully.

In unstable pseudarthroses, therefore, a discussion of treatment resolves itself first into considerations of early operation to prevent or correct displacement. Displacement contributes greatly to the difficulties of repair, if not rendering this impossible. It is equally important that we recognize at an early stage those for whom early operation is neither necessary nor rewarding. Secondly, we must consider the techniques available for alleviation of the total handicap in older children with established malformations. These children may suffer from persistent instability because of procrastination in performing an early operation when this was indicated, or from failure of such an operation, or because the anomaly precludes repair. Leg length discrepancy will be considerable in these and in some of those with natural or surgically contrived stability. This, in practice, now becomes the dominating problem. Lastly, and throughout, we must with the aid of the prosthetist select the appliance suitable not only to the nature of the deformity but also to the age and needs of the patient.

Early surgical treatment

The decision for or against early operation should be taken at about one year of age to anticipate independent walking and the consequent risk of displacement at a point of instability. Children with defects of the proximal femur are not unduly delayed in walking for at this age shortening is compensated for by a tip-toe gait.

Contra-indications

Operation is unnecessary at this age when instability is absent or not expected to develop. Such patients include those with simple congenital short femur with or without coxa vara and those with proximal dysplasia who exhibit the radiological features already described, which suggest that stability in this area will be maintained. The second contra-indicated group are those in whom it will not be possible to restore stability with mobility proximally — i.e. serious defects involving subtotal loss of the femur in whom lack of the acetabular cup is evidence of absence of the femoral head. Thirdly, the potential benefit is doubtful in severe bilateral proximal deficiencies for the ultimate shortening will inevitably require bilateral extension prostheses and the maintenance of mobility proximally will outweigh other considerations especially if knee fusion is desirable later.

Lastly, we must remember as in all congenital malformations arising during the stage of embryonic differentiation that there is the possibility that some other possibly life-threatening disorder may be present which will dominate our principles of management.

Indications

Early exploration is recommended for those who are not included in the above categories, namely proximal deficiency with a poor prognosis for spontaneous stabilization, associated dislocation of the hip with an otherwise good prognosis, and indolent subtrochanteric defects liable to develop pseudarthrosis.

There will inevitably be some in whom there is uncertainty about the likely outcome. For example there are those in whom the signs by which we decide between a good and poor prognosis for subsequent stability are less definite than usual and there are the rare examples of doubtful spontaneous union in a sub-trochanteric pseudarthrosis. It is then probably better to explore the hip than run the risk of displacement in an area of persisting instability (*Figure 1.15*).

Surgical techniques

Approach The hip is approached from the front by a long Smith-Petersen incision extending down to the distal third of the short femur. Fixed flexion of the hip adds an element of apparent to the true shortening and in the initial

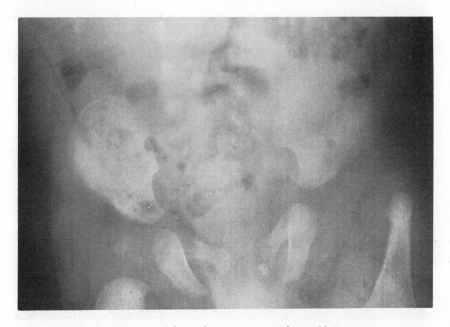

Figure 1.15. (a) In infancy the signs suggest a favourable outcome

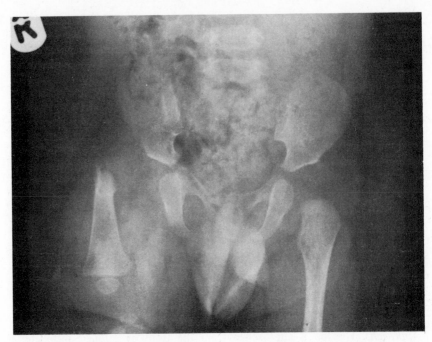

Figure 1.15. (b) The proximal femur is becoming pointed

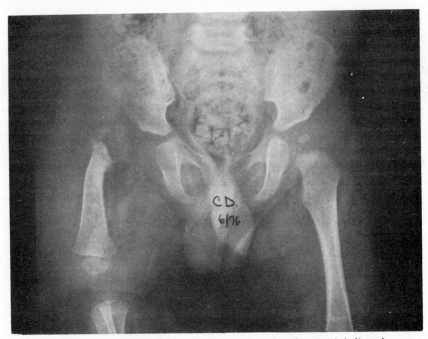

Figure 1.15. (c) The pattern is now uncertain and exploration is indicated

steps the approach may be somewhat cramped. However, the musculature will be found to be anatomically normal and as the origin of gluteus medius and the muscular and fascial components of tensor fascia femoris are released so flexion and external rotation deformities yield and access improves. The target is the head, neck and trochanteric area but it is simpler to work upwards from below exposing the femoral shaft distally than to engage the target directly. Once the shaft is exposed, vastus lateralis is dissected from the bone as far as its origin in front of the intertrochanteric line. Gluteus medius and minimus are further mobilized from the joint capsule which may then be opened in the line of the neck with, if necessary, a transverse extension parallel to the acetabulum. Any residual fixed flexion or external rotation may now be released by detachment of the origins of rectus femoris and gluteus medius as far posteriorly as possible with division of the psoas tendon. The anatomy of the malformation in its various manifestations is now displayed and further steps will be dictated by these findings.

(a) *Continuity of the femur with dislocation of the hip*

This is very rare and I have experience of only one example. Both the acetabulum and femoral head were comparable to those seen in ordinary congenital dislocation but the anteversion angle was very greatly increased and soft tissue shortening was considerable. Consequently reduction could only be effected with unacceptable tension and the patella pointing backwards. The reduction was secured by

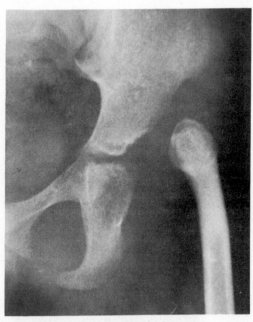

Figure 1.16. (a) The hip is dislocated but the tip of the femur is bulbous and the acetabulum relatively well formed

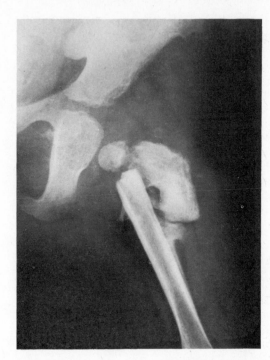

Figure 1.16.(b) After open re-duction, and osteotomy with shortening

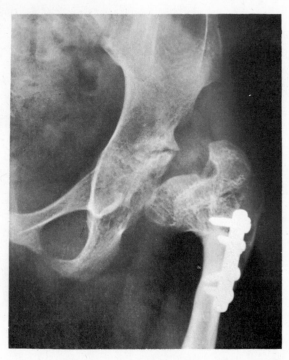

Figure 1.16.(c) The out-come six years later

capsular suture and Kirschner wire and the femur divided to correct rotation and tension by allowing overlapping of the fragments without internal fixation. Reduction was maintained and stability restored with a useful though limited range of movement (*Figure 1.16*).

(b) *Persisting subtrochanteric pseudarthrosis*

This presents no problem for it may be stabilized by an intramedullary nail and union may be encouraged by onlaying cancellous bone readily obtained from the adjacent ilium (*Figure 1.9*).

(c) *Trochanteric and cervical pseudarthroses*

These may be displaced so that a considerable coxa vara deformity develops with the head lying well below the trochanters or relative stability may have preserved a near normal configuration. These should be managed differently.

(1) Stable pseudarthroses without deformity may be transfixed undisturbed in the manner of a Smith-Petersen pin by a cortical graft taken from the fibula. Cancellous bone is then laid on the surfaces of the defect. Six weeks later an oblique intertrochanteric osteotomy is performed displacing the lower fragment medially and into abduction to reinforce the area of weakness and convert any residual varus to valgus thus reducing the stress imposed on the weak area when walking begins (Lloyd-Roberts and Stone, 1963) (*Figure 1.17*).

(2) Unstable pseudarthroses with displacement. In these circumstances the operation described above has been unsuccessful in my hands, because the gap to be bridged is too great, the transfixing graft is in a mechanically unsound position, and the displacement osteotomy is less easily apposed to the pseudarthrosis. Furthermore, I have on one occasion found a double pseudarthrosis at trochanteric and cervical levels with an isolated cartilaginous segment between them, which inevitably affected the outcome. There are three possibilities: to abandon the operation; to perform femoropelvic arthrodesis (*see later*); or to attempt to obtain fusion between the femoral shaft and head after excision of the pseudarthrosis and the neck as far as the capital growth plate (King, 1969). It would seem reasonable to attempt the third proposition, for even if this fails the alternatives are not compromised. The head is partially enucleated and the cartilaginous tip of the trochanter excised to bleeding bone which is then inserted into the concavity within the head in full abduction which achieves compression. The fragments are held by a Kirschner wire which is run up the femur, through the head, and into the pelvis. The abductors are advanced and attached to the shaft distally. If successful this operation will ensure stability with some limited movement but deformity requiring a secondary corrective osteotomy may be necessary (*Figure 1.18*).

(d) *Unnecessary and secondary operations*

Because we are unable to see pseudarthroses within scantily ossified cartilage we can only suspect their presence by inference. Sometimes exploration will not disclose a pseudarthrosis. However the issues at stake are so important that this

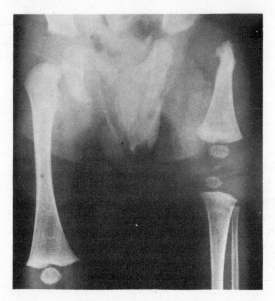

Figure 1.17. (a) The tip of the femur is spiked suggesting that pseudarthrosis is present

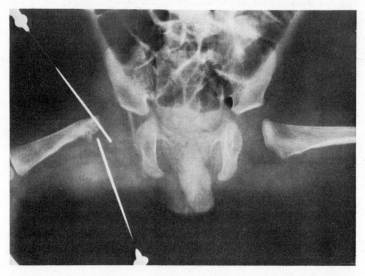

Figure 1.17. (b) In abduction there is no displacement. Stability is present.

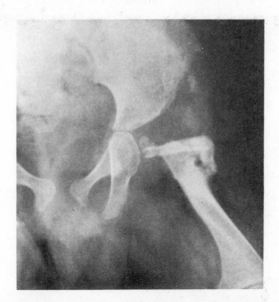

Figure 1.17. (c) The fibula graft in position. The head is visible and the osteotomy has been performed

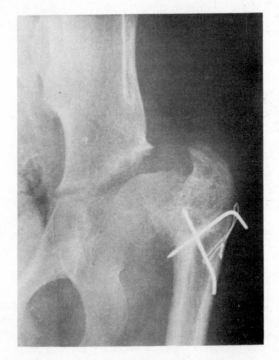

Figure 1.17. (d) The outcome at the age of seven

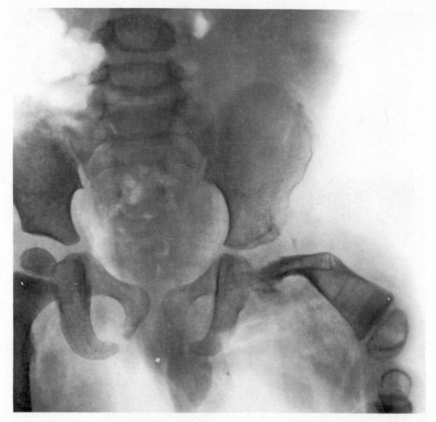

Figure 1.18. (a) The femoral shaft has been inserted into the head and an osteotomy performed

is a justifiable error when there is uncertainty in the interpretation of early radiographs. (*Figure 1.15*).

That the first operation offers the best prospect of success is a well supported maxim of surgery. It is particularly true in proximal femoral dysplasia. Secondary operations are made much more difficult by reason of residual scar tissue and further distortion of the anatomy. It may still be possible to obtain union between the femoral shaft and head but too often the head has become ankylosed to the acetabulum and then this operation has no advantage over the simpler femoro-pelvic arthrodesis.

(e) *Miscellaneous observations*

Hip and knee flexion deformities are common and, if persistent, prejudice prosthetic fitting. Most respond to stretching but some are severe and obstinate. If operation is indicated hip deformity may be corrected at the time of recon-struction, otherwise operation may be necessary for this purpose alone. The knee also may resist correction and require posterior capsulotomy. Knee and hip

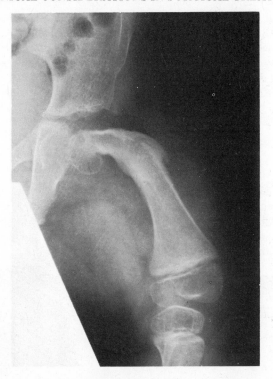

Figure 1.18. (b) The appearance seven years later

flexion deformities perpetuate one another so that correction of one aids the resolution of the other. Thus, if the knee will straighten sufficiently for the application of plaster tubes to both legs with a cross bar and the child lies prone, hip flexion will usually improve.

Acute angular deformities of the femoral shaft tend to straighten rapidly but are points of weakness; they may fracture, but union is to be anticipated.

In the beginning it is prudent to preserve working stock and it is for example, unwise to perform Syme's amputation at this stage. The foot may be at first contained within an extension prosthesis without disadvantage and amputation considered later if the Van Nes rotation-plasty is to be rejected or the extra length deemed unhelpful.

Lastly, avoid too much scientific zeal, for a positive answer to questions about drugs in pregnancy will add unnecessary anxiety to the mother's distress. There is time later.

Late surgical treatment

We may, in general, define late treatment as that which is applied to those children with unilateral malformations in whom the opportunity to retain stability with movement has been overlooked or has failed, together with those who by reason of the severity of the malformation (lacking femoral head and acetabulum with perhaps absence of half or more of the femur) are not amenable to repair. Of course it may be possible to perform femorocapital fusion in some of the first group but in most we must now resort to operations in which we accept the loss of either stability or movement at the hip joint.

We must also consider secondary operations in those cases with retained hip function, the correction of coxa vara, the possibilities of leg equalization in simple short femur and the indications for amputation of the foot.

(a) *Proximal deficiency with hip instability*

We may consider stabilization of the hip or knee, substituting the ankle for the knee, and replacing the femur with the tibia.

(1) *Stabilization operations*   Arthrodesis of the femur to the pelvis, arthrodesis of the knee and, when the femur is completely absent, tibiopelvic fusion, all merit discussion.

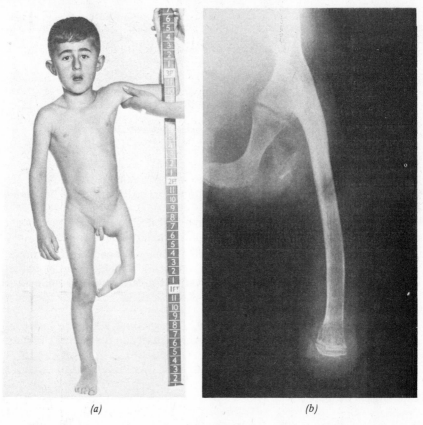

(a)   *(b)*

Figure 1.19. (a) Fusion of the tibia to the pelvis when the femur is completely absent. (b) The absent acetabulum confirms that the head is absent. The rounded structure is the tibial epiphysis

Although I have once performed tibiopelvic fusion with subsequent Syme's amputation I doubt whether this confers any benefit over Syme's amputation and the use of the tibia as an above-knee stump, thus retaining mobility in spite of instability at the tibiopelvic articulation (*Figure 1.19*).

The indication for knee or hip fusion is much the same but the rationale is different. When the ankle joint is or is likely to become proximal to the normal

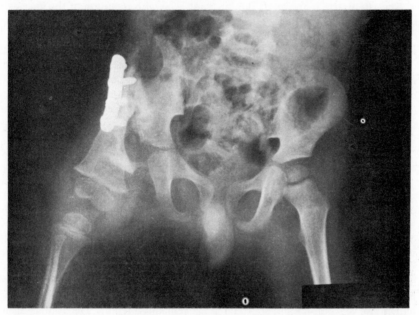

Figure 1.20. Fusion of the femur to the pelvis with proximal displacement of the knee joint

knee, rotation-plasty to produce ankle–knee substitution is contra-indicated (*see below, Figure 1.21*). A further contra-indication is an abnormal foot which may be expected when tibial dysplasia is associated with the femoral. In these circumstances we must perforce consider stabilization at one or other level. Even in those cases suitable for rotation-plasty arthrodesis is regarded by many as preferable to this operation.

Arthrodesis of the knee lengthens and stabilizes the limb to give a longer lever to which an 'above-knee' prosthesis is applied. It enables any remaining knee flexion or other deformity (especially valgus) to be corrected, and depends for mobility upon the unstable hip. The foot is redundant and is removed at the ankle joint. The pelvifemoral muscles ensure that there is good control of the stump.

Ideally the length of stump should be such that a knee hinge may be included in the prosthesis in spite of the technical difficulties posed to the prosthetist. If this is not contemplated, length is somewhat less significant. In either event, however, it would seem undesirable to injure the growth plates in a young child, for excessive shortening will reduce the effectiveness of both hinged and unhinged prostheses. This risk is increased when a wedge has to be cut from largely carti-laginous epiphyses to correct deformity. Furthermore, sound union is favoured by epiphyseal ossification so that it would seem preferable to delay this operation until maturity is approaching, when length may be adjusted to prosthetic require-ments and compression may be used. If for some reason it is necessary to intervene earlier, compression is of course contra-indicated but the growth plates may be preserved if a centrally placed intramedullary nail is used.

The alternative is fusion at the hip joint level with retention of the knee as a stable hinge, a method which has interested me almost to the exclusion of the other (*Figure 1.20*). The tibia, after removal of the foot, becomes the prosthetic lever, but we now have a stable, partially mobile and well controlled proximal component. The femoral and tibial growth plates are not at risk so that operation may be carried out at any age for the lower femur and pelvis are well ossified ensuring that union is rapid. Control of the stump is assured for the muscles serving the knee are normal. This method may have a special appeal when the femur is represented by no more than the distal supracondylar segment and the femoral head and acetabulum are absent.

Technical considerations include the method of pelvifemoral fixation and the relationship of the knee joint to the pelvis. Following removal of any remaining cartilaginous model proximally, the ossified distal femur is decorticated on the medial side and applied to the similarly treated pelvic wall above the acetabulum or its remnant. Contact is secured by screws transfixing femur and ilium, with or without a plate. The position of the knee is all important. The length and shape of the femur should be adjusted so that the knee hinge lies as near the pelvis as possible, in slight pelvifemoral abduction and some flexion. Flexion enables the tibial stump to move forwards ahead of the trunk in walking and this is augmented by the spontaneous development of hyperextension at the knee when this is established. Growth continues so that the knee will move distally and in one patient we are considering shortening the remaining femur. The foot is again redundant and should be removed.

I have performed this operation four times and although none has reached skeletal maturity the early results justify modest satisfaction.

(2) *Rotation-plasty (Van Nes, 1950)* This ingenious operation aims to use the ankle as a knee by rotating the tibia through 180°, the reversed foot being placed in the socket of the prosthesis (*Figure 1.21*). This should not be confused with the tibial turn-up plasty designed by the same author to replace the femur removed for malignant disease. It is tempting to consider turn-up plasty when the femur is congenitally absent or represented by condyles alone and I have known this possibility to be seriously discussed. Unfortunately in such patients the acetabulum is usually absent so that there is no natural stabilizing point for the medial malleolus. Furthermore the tibia will migrate proximally with time and achieve the same objective.

The rotation-plasty however has a definite role in management. My personal experience is limited to three patients which is enough to alert me to the numerous problems inherent in the operation. These, however, are not insuperable. Pre-requisites are a normal foot and ankle either lying at the level of the opposite knee or distal to it. Further shortening by resection at the knee with concomitant arthrodesis then achieves this level. Instability of the hip is not a contra-indication. The operation itself is simple and vascular complications are not a significant hazard. Failure is not a disaster for the foot may be amputated and knee or pelvifemoral arthrodesis performed.

Rotation is combined with some tibial shortening to relax the soft tissues and in some cases to align the ankle with the opposite knee. The osteotomy is fixed with a plate. If knee arthrodesis is contemplated some rotation may be obtained

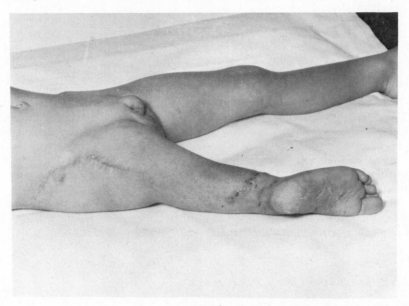

Figure 1.21. Van Nes operation. The tibia has been rotated and the foot now points backwards

at this level to reduce the tibial torsion. The ankle and foot should be fully mobile with good muscle control and at the end of the operation the plane should be transverse as in a normal knee.

The major problem is derotation towards normal tibial alignment, the risk being directly proportional to the age of the patient. Delaying operation to beyond the age of twelve not only reduces this risk but allows more time for consideration of the indications. Secondary problems include the child's dislike of the somewhat grotesque appearance of the rotated ankle within the prosthesis and uncertainty about the functional performance as opposed to its performance on the examination couch.

Some of these aspects have been discussed recently in a valuable paper by Kostuik *et al.* (1975).

(b) *Proximal deficiency with hip stability and mobility*

Whether this has arisen naturally or as a result of successful early surgery there is no urgency about deciding upon the next step. At first most children will walk

31

on tip-toe without a prosthesis and this is to be encouraged for it will not only absolve us from the need to provide at least one and possibly more extension prostheses but also stimulate the foot and ankle to develop equinus deformity, so that ultimate fitting of the prosthesis is simplified. An extension prosthesis incorporating the foot is the method of choice during early childhood and only later should we consider arthrodesis of the knee with sacrifice of the foot or rotation-plasty with preservation of the foot for the reasons and indications already mentioned.

(c) *Congenital short femur*

Provided that there is no coxa vara and the tibia is normal the final shortening is unlikely to exceed 2–2½ in (~5–6½ cm) which should usually be accepted. The alternatives are leg lengthening and contralateral shortening. The problems of lengthening are discussed below but in considering shortening it should be remembered that these children often grow into short adults so that operations such as epiphysiodesis should be avoided. At skeletal maturity, however, the situation will be clarified and if the patient wishes, a segment may be resected from the opposite femur.

It has already been mentioned that this variety is very commonly seen in association with an absent fibula and short tibia. Severe shortening will indicate Syme's amputation in most of these (Hootnick *et al.*, 1977).

(d) *Congenital short femur with coxa vara*

The two patterns of coxa vara with which we are concerned have been described earlier and require separate discussion. First the persistent pseudarthrosis (Type IIIB) with subsequent displacement (IIIC) or even disintegration (IIID) presents us with opportunities to intervene usefully at each stage. If coxa vara with a wide 'epiphyseal plate' is recognized early as a dangerous situation, operation may prevent displacement. Wide-abduction intertrochanteric osteotomy with displacement beneath the femoral neck, or even wider subtrochanteric osteotomy to convert the vertically disposed zone of pre-pseudarthrosis to the horizontal, is the first essential step.

If displacement has already occurred or the neck is becoming attenuated and stippled in appearance, it is necessary to reinforce the femoral neck with a split fibular or tibial graft in the manner of a Smith-Petersen pin (*Figure 1.17*). Further security is provided by metal fixation parallel to the graft. The implant used will vary from a Kirschner wire to a Knowle's pin depending upon the age of the child. Abduction and medial displacement osteotomy follows at a second stage. Amstutz and Wilson (1962) have discussed both this problem and the variation discussed below in great depth and advocate an ingenious intertrochanteric interlocking osteotomy of which I have no experience but which is immediately appealing.

When disintegration and wide displacement has evolved we must still attempt to restore stability by femoral shaft-head fusion as described earlier.

The second variety characterized by a modest degree of cervical coxa vara, lateral bowing of the femur, bullet-shaped head and, in some, acetabular dysplasia and subluxation, presents a totally different problem (*Figure 1.11*). The neck-shaft angle is stable, does not progress, and the degree of varus does not warrant correction in its own right. Abduction osteotomy would be rational only if it is believed that we could thereby prevent the development of acetabular dysplasia by reducing the pressure between the top of the misshapen head and the acetabulum. This implies that acetabular changes are due more to this pressure than congenital factors. While this remains unproven, restoring a valgus inclination to the femoral neck will aggravate the tendency to subluxation if dysplasia develops spontaneously and it is therefore best avoided.

If acetabular growth is deficient we must consider its reinforcement by acetabuloplasty, shelf, or Chiari osteotomy, depending upon the age of the patient and the degree of subluxation. Otherwise it is prudent to withhold surgical treatment.

(e) Leg lengthening

This has been mentioned as a possibility in simple femoral shortening but is more appropriate to shortening with coxa vara when the discrepancy may be of the order of 4 in (~10 cm). Allan (1948) has succeeded in 4 patients with simple shortening but our experience has been discouraging in 5. Elongation and union were uncomplicated but failure to restore normal bone architecture at the point of union was followed by fracture, delayed union and loss of correction in 4. We have therefore abandoned this operation in this context. In this we are supported by Amstutz and Wilson (1962) who were discouraged from leg lengthening by a zone of marked sclerosis in the area of proposed bone section.

(f) Amputation

Disarticulation at the knee and below-knee ablation with its attendant problems during further growth hold no attraction in this condition when Syme's amputation meets all our needs. With the possible exception of pelvifemoral arthrodesis with a tibia long enough to satisfy the prosthetist, there is no need to amputate in early childhood. This is in contrast to the indication when congenital tibial shortening predominates over femoral. It is better to wait until a choice can be made between a permanent extension prosthesis preserving the foot, rotation-plasty incorporating the foot, and arthrodesis of the knee which indicates its removal.

There are two technical points which merit attention in childhood. First, growth should usually be preserved and the line of section is therefore at the level of the tibial articular cartilage with appropriate resection of the malleoli to this level. Secondly, there is a tendency for the heel flap to migrate posteriorly especially if anterior tibial bowing is present. The flap should therefore be secured by the addition of cross-strapping and a transfixing Kirschner wire into the tibia. Tibial osteotomy, so far, has not been necessary.

REFERENCES

Aitken, G. T. (1969). Proximal femoral focal deficiency – definition, classification and management. In *Proximal Femoral Focal Deficiency: A Congenital Anomaly*. A symposium held in Washington, D.C., on June 13th, 1968. p. 1. Ed. G. T. Aitken. Washington D.C. : National Academy of Sciences

Allan, F. G. (1948). Bone lengthening. *J. Bone Jt Surg.* **30B**, 490

Amstutz, H. C. (1969). The morphology, natural history, and treatment of proximal femoral focal deficiencies. In *Proximal Femoral Focal Deficiency: A Congenital Anomaly*. A symposium held in Washington D.C., on June 13th 1968. p. 50. Ed. G. T. Aitken. Washington D.C. : National Academy of Sciences

Amstutz, H. C., and Wilson, P. D. (1962). Dysgenesis of the proximal femur (coxa vara) and its surgical management. *J. Bone Jt Surg.* **44A**, 1

Blockey, N. J. (1969). Observations on infantile coxa vara. *J. Bone Jt Surg.* **51B**, 106

Duraiswami, P. K. (1952). Experimental causation of congenital skeletal defects and its significance in orthopaedic surgery. *J. Bone Jt Surg.* **34B**, 646

Fixsen, J. A. and Lloyd-Roberts, G. C. (1974). The natural history and early treatment of proximal femoral dysplasia. *J. Bone Jt Surg.* **56B**, 86

Golding, F. C. (1948). Congenital coxa vara. *J. Bone Jt Surg.* **30B**, 161

Hootnick, D., Boyd, N.A., Fixsen, J. A., and Lloyd-Roberts, G. C. (1977). The natural history and management of congenital short tibia (fibular dysplasia or congenital absence of the fibula). *J. Bone Jt Surg.* **59B**. In press

King, R. E. (1969). Some concepts of proximal femoral focal deficiency. In *Proximal Femoral Focal Deficiency: A Congenital Anomaly*. A symposium held in Washington D.C. on June 13th, 1968. p. 23. Ed. G. T. Aitken. Washington D.C. : National Academy of Sciences

Kostuik, J. P., Gillespie, R., Hall, J. E. and Sheila Hubbard (1975). Van Nes rotational osteotomy for treatment of proximal femoral focal deficiency and congenital short femur. *J. Bone Jt Surg.* **57A**, 1039

Kučera, J., Lenz, W. and Maier, W. (1965). Malformations of the lower limbs and the caudal part of the spinal column in children of diabetic mothers. *Germ. med. Mon.* **10**, 393

Lloyd-Roberts, G. C. and Stone, K. H. (1963). Congenital hypoplasia of the upper femur. *J. Bone Jt Surg.* **45B**, 557

Morgan, J. D., and Somerville, E. W. (1960). Normal and abnormal growth at the upper end of the femur. *J. Bone Jt Surg.* **42B**, 264

Ring, P. A. (1959). Congenital short femur. Simple femoral hypoplasia. *J. Bone Jt Surg.* **41B**, 73

Ring, P. A. (1961). Congenital abnormalities of the femur. *Archs. Dis. Childh.* **36**, 410

Van Nes, C. P. (1950). Rotation-plasty for congenital defects of the femur. Making use of the ankle of the shortened limb to control the knee joint of a prosthesis. *J. Bone Jt Surg.* **32B**, 12

2

Congenital Dislocation of the Hip and Associated Conditions

G. C. Lloyd- Roberts

There are four distinct manifestations of this malformation. In infancy we must consider unstable hips and pelvic obliquity and in the older child dislocation and subluxation. Pelvic obliquity is less well delineated than the others and while there is evidence to suggest that it should be included in the syndrome it is as yet uncertain whether general observations about the nature and cause of dislocation and its subdivisions are applicable to it.

GENERAL OBSERVATIONS UPON CAUSE AND NATURE

The basic facts are well known. The ratio of girls to boys is 6:1, of unilateral to bilateral 1:2, and of winter to summer births 1.5:1. Racial influence is strong for some seem immune whereas in North-West Europe the incidence is about 1.5 per 1 000 live births with breech births and first-born predominating. Genetically the risk to a succeeding sibling of an affected child depends upon the presence of dislocation in one parent. If present this risk is 36 per cent; if absent, 6 per cent (Wynne-Davies, 1970).

Few congenital abnormalities are exclusively congenital or environmental in origin and hip dislocation is no exception. We must therefore consider a multifactorial aetiology which includes the genetic influence which predominantly affects the acetabulum and the environmental dependent upon intra-uterine factors, and joint laxity which may be either congenital or secondary to hormonal disturbance.

Wynne-Davies (1970) has carefully examined the relative influence of acetabular dysplasia and joint laxity by comparing the incidence of both in babies with neonatal instability and in those in whom the diagnosis of dislocation was made later. It seemed probable that identification of the factors which determine spontaneous correction of neonatal instability or the converse would illuminate our uncertainty. The dislocated group displayed a significantly higher proportion of radiological acetabular dysplasia among their parents than the unstable and the incidence of this increased in direct relation to the severity of the child's dysplasia. Furthermore these patients with late dislocation could be separated from the unstable in other respects. There was no predominance of first-born nor winter-born babies, the sex ratio approaches unity and unilateral dislocation was relatively uncommon. Wilkinson and Carter (1960) have also drawn attention to the high incidence of contralateral acetabular dysplasia in 'unilateral' dislocations. Wynne-Davies has also shown that delay in femoral capital ossification is significant in dislocation but that this does not occur in those with instability corrected in infancy. There seems, therefore, persuasive evidence that acetabular dysplasia is an aetiological factor inherited as a multiple gene system of particular importance in those patients with true dislocation diagnosed after infancy.

Joint laxity may be familial (Carter and Wilkinson, 1964) or possibly hormonal and related to relaxin as an anomaly of oestrogen metabolism (Andren and Borglin, 1961). Although the influence of joint laxity of either variety is seen in neonatal and late cases, its impact is greatest in the neonatal group. The nature of joint laxity is uncertain for hormonal assay has not confirmed a transitory state of imbalance which might operate in the neonatal period. A generalized minor defect in connective tissue is a possibility for laxity is associated with a higher rate of other connective tissue anomalies than a random sample of the population. Wynne-Davies (1970) has pointed out that laxity is not demonstrable in the first week of life but reaches its maximum incidence at about two years, after which it diminishes to under 1 per cent of children by the age of 12. Although a higher proportion of children with late dislocation were more lax jointed than a control population this difference is accentuated in neonatal instability when it is associated with a higher incidence in first-degree relatives. Wilkinson (1963) has discussed fully the possible significance of laxity at different stages of intra-uterine and postnatal life. He has also studied the effects of splinting the hind limbs of rabbits (to simulate the breech position) with and without hormone-induced joint laxity. In combination these caused a high incidence of dislocation which did not develop when the challenges were applied separately.

We have, therefore, evidence to show that both primary acetabular dysplasia and joint laxity may be factors of aetiological importance at different ages and in varying degree. It is evident, however, that when present in isolation neither will necessarily cause dislocation and we must therefore seek for some trigger mechanism which may well be the result of abnormal intra-uterine environment or fetal posture. Denis Browne (1936), for example, noted the association between a calcaneus foot and dislocation of the hip on the same side. This observation is valid and suggests that an upward thrust upon the foot by a tight uterus may dislocate the hip. Again, Dunn (1969) has shown that the left hip may be compressed against the sacral promontory in the breech position thus suggesting an explanation for the association between left-sided dislocations (which predominate) and breech presentation. First-born babies are at greater risk and we may therefore postulate a tight uterus and diminished liquor restricting fetal movement and preventing cephalic version.

Restriction of free movement is seen in other conditions which are also associated with breech presentation and hip dislocation possibly because some factor prevents the fetus from rotating from breech to cephalic before delivery. The physiological mechanism of this is uncertain. In arthrogryposis, weakness and deformity combine and breech presentation with dislocation is frequently seen;

lack of liquor in oligohydramnios is similarly associated (Dunn, 1969). Myelo-meningocele is the more familiar example when differential paralysis favouring dislocation also inhibits fetal movement. Lastly, congenital hypotonia of severe degree may behave similarly. These children have joint laxity in addition to weakness thereby bringing us back to one of the prime factors. Wilkinson (1963) has discussed the association between laxity, breech presentation or malposition and dislocation and with some ingenuity suggests a mechanism by which dis-location may occur when the legs are either extended and medially rotated or semiflexed and laterally rotated.

When considering the primary anatomical malformations we are immediately in difficulty when we attempt to distinguish between these and the secondary effects of an established dislocation. It is these secondary structural adaptations which we see when operating on the older child. We do not know, for example, whether femoral or acetabular anteversion and anterior acetabular deficiency are primary or secondary. Some features, however, are clearly secondary such as a false acetabulum, infolding of capsule over the transverse ligament of the ligamentum teres and probably the labrum (limbus) which is inverted in dis-location and flattened in subluxation. Furthermore, there is probably a difference between the pathological anatomy in congenital neonatal instability (which usually recovers spontaneously) and congenital dislocation, so that autopsy studies may be misleading when the provenance is insecure.

McKibbin (1970) was fortunate to obtain a specimen from a full-term baby who died of cerebral haemorrhage shortly after birth. It is notable that the presentation was by the breech with extended legs. We are fortunate in that this specimen was dissected with great thoroughness, to disclose no more than redundant capsule, elongation of the ligamentum teres and relative psoas-shortening in extension. It must be emphasized however that the hips, although dislocated, were easily reducible and should probably, therefore, be classified as examples of neonatal instability. We do not know if spontaneous correction would have occurred or whether, if untreated, irreducible dislocation would have followed. In this connection the negative findings may be as significant as the positive for a malformation of one or more of the apparently normal structures may be the factor which determines an unfavourable outcome. There was, for example, no evidence of primary acetabular dysplasia nor indeed of any other inherent structural abnormality such as anteversion. Further dissections of normal hips have shown that congruous stability is less secure at birth than in intra-uterine life and in children over the age of two years (Ralis and McKibbin, 1973). This, incidentally, is the age from which joint laxity tends to diminish. Although others have reported neonatal acetabular deficiency (Stanisavljevic and Mitchell, 1963), this does not necessarily convict the acetabulum for the dis-location may have become irreducible during intra-uterine life for some uncon-nected reason and the acetabular deficiency may be secondary to this. Indeed, it is not uncommon to notice a well developed false acetabulum on the radiograph even before walking begins when a dislocation, although detected early, does not respond to reduction by non-operative means.

Le Damany (1908) first proposed that a difference in orientation between acetabular and femoral anteversion might be significant. When incompatible a state of instability may arise which Le Damany quantified as the instability index. This was not present in McKibbin's specimen for both measurements were within the normal range. The concept of acetabular anteversion is, however, one of great practical importance in the older child in whom it is commonly found at operation. A method of measurement applicable either before or during operation so far eludes us but we are at present investigating the problem by using the infantiscope which is a radiological screening technique in which the child is rotated while the tube remains stationary.

If we turn again to the positive findings of elongation of the ligamentum teres and capsular redundancy, the implication is that displacement was present during uterine life for they could hardly have developed during the few hours that the child lived. Neither is incompatible with spontaneous correction nor with progressive dislocation. Stability was however related to position. Flexion in the neutral position was the least stable position, whereas abduction and internal rotation tightened the capsule and improved stability. It is perhaps surprising that flexion is undesirable for we are cautioned against extension because of the risk of levering the femoral head forwards out of the acetabulum. In fact the hip was more stable in extension which again tightens the capsule whereas flexion relaxes it. This observation is not as paradoxical as it seems for it is not natural extension but forcible extension that must be avoided (Somerville, 1953; Salter, 1966). The psoas was, in fact, short and when divided there was no increased instability on forced extension. The normal baby has some fixed flexion of the hips so this was probably to be expected for, as McKibbin says, if such a contracture were commonly responsible this would imply that the dislocation was postnatal and so unlikely to be associated with the changes in the capsule and ligamentum teres already present at birth.

Both hips were affected in McKibbin's patient but we must not necessarily assume that the cause and nature of dislocation is the same in unilateral dislocations as perhaps we too readily tend to do. In clinical practice they are certainly very different. It is more difficult to obtain a good result in one hip of a pair than in a strictly unilateral dislocation by either conservative or surgical methods. The differences are particularly apparent at operation in the older child, for open reduction of a unilateral dislocation at the age of 3 years is often simple with little to distinguish it from a similar operation performed at 1 year. In contrast, bilateral dislocations in the older child disclose anatomical abnormalities of a degree which may be technically testing to the surgeon. These include acetabular insufficiency, anteversion with pear-shaped malformation and femoral-head deformity with subcapital capsular attachment. These differences in the anatomy between unilateral and bilateral dislocations explored at the same age suggest the possibility of differences in aetiology and developmental potential. The obvious, if perhaps too simplistic, explanation is that unilateral dislocations are predominantly environmental in origin whereas the genetic factors are paramount in the bilateral.

If there is an essential lesion which is present at birth and determines whether the hip is irreducibly dislocated or merely in a state of transitory instability, this still eludes us. It seems most likely that one or more factors such as familial laxity and acetabular dysplasia combine with an abnormal fetal posture and intra-uterine environment to lead sometimes to a final common path which is prenatal dislocation. Alternatively, if these combined influences are less potent they may set the stage for postnatal dislocation when neonatal instability, which does not resolve spontaneously, persists unrecognized and untreated.

NEONATAL INSTABILITY OF THE HIP

Although neonatal screening for hip-joint instability remains of considerable contemporary significance, the principles were established by Poser in 1879 and advocated by Putti in 1927. Ortolani (1937) was responsible for a renewal of interest but his method aimed at detection at between three and nine months of age. By 1950, about half of the children born in Sweden were examined as newborns (Palmen, 1961) and in 1952 Von Rosen (1962) began his well-known work in Malmö. Barlow (1962) should be credited with initiating and stimulating interest in Britain. He also developed the screening test which bears his name and which is now the generally favoured method.

Barlow's method is well known and will detect two varieties of instability. With the pelvis secured with one hand the middle finger of the other presses forwards on the great trochanter as the hip is abducted. If displaced backwards the head slips forward into the acetabulum with an audible, palpable and often visible clunk or jolt. If unstable but reduced, pressure in a backward direction by the thumb will dislocate it backwards. The term 'click' is frequently used to describe the clunk, jolt or jerk of a positive finding. This is unfortunate for clicks are commonplace and of no significance. When a true clunk is present it may represent either reduction of habitual displacement or dislocation of a hip whose stability is insecure (Finlay, Maudsley and Busfield, 1967) and it is natural to assume the first variety to be the more significant but in practice further development runs parallel in both.

Neonatal screening should not be confined to the detection of the clunk but extended to determine whether there is any loss of abduction in flexion and real or apparent shortening when, with hips and knees flexed, the levels of the femoral condyles are compared. This is an essential step for in babies with pelvic obliquity we will not elicit a clunk and the clunk is rarely present when intra-uterine dislocation has become established and irreducible at birth. It may reasonably be suggested that some of those dislocations which present later, having escaped detection on neonatal examination for a clunk, would have been identified if limited abduction had been sought. Similarly, some late subluxations may well have arisen as a result of undetected pelvic obliquity.

Opinions differ about the value of radiographs at this age. When abduction is limited they are certainly important for distinguishing between dislocation and pelvic obliquity, but when instability is present the findings will depend upon whether the hip is displaced or not when the radiographs are taken. Furthermore, interpretation, particularly when positioning is suspect, may be difficult and thus misleading especially if diagnosis depends upon the estimation of acetabular angles. If radiological examination is favoured, Von Rosen's projection is probably that most commonly employed. The legs with knees extended are abducted to 45° and medially rotated and a line projected in the axis of the femur. This should normally cross the lateral margin of the acetabulum but if the hip is dislocated it crosses the anterior superior iliac spine. False positive and negative readings are frequent. MacKenzie (1972) reported 70 per cent false negatives in infancy when correlated with a positive Barlow sign. Although the value of radiographs is questionable in infancy there is no doubt about their importance when the baby is re-examined at the age of three months or later.

It is essential to consider the value of neonatal screening with a sense of perspective. Such an approach is hampered by emotive, political, journalistic and medicolegal issues, but nevertheless an attempt must be made. In 1962, Von Rosen and Barlow reported independently upon large numbers of babies whose hips were examined in the neonatal period. Their success in both detection and treatment encouraged the uncritical to believe that late presentations of congenital dislocations would disappear, for diagnosis seemed to be simple and splinting in abduction consistently successful. Such was the enthusiasm that the Department of Health, perhaps somewhat ill-advisedly and prematurely, issued a brochure which implied among other things, that failure to achieve comparable results constituted a malpractice which was little short of negligence. Nevertheless, those seeing large numbers of children continued to treat congenital dislocation presenting over the age of one year in children who had been examined with negative results in early infancy. What had gone wrong?

There were and are several basic reasons for failure to eradicate established dislocation. First, there is the human element. This task is usually delegated to the obstetric or paediatric house officer who is characteristically overworked. He will have to examine about 1000 babies to elicit a clunk 6 times and being well educated in those matters he will know that of these less than 1 will, if undetected, fail to stabilize spontaneously. His enthusiasm may falter. Secondly, obsessed with the sign of the clunk he and his teachers may well have forgotten the greater significance of limitation of abduction in flexion.

The next problem is one of organization and the obstetric environment. Babies born at home or in small maternity units are likely to be at a disadvantage. Similarly, in large centres of population or in dispersed rural communities the organization of total screening is difficult to enforce. In contrast, smaller towns with relatively static populations in which all the babies are born in one institution offer the greatest prospect of success. This is specially so when all primigravida and those suspected of being at risk to obstetric complications are segregated. It is under such conditions that a skilled examiner may be available to examine all babies with suspected instability and all those at special risk, be it familial or positional such as breech presentations. It was, in fact, under these circumstances that Von Rosen in Malmö (1968) and Mitchell in Edinburgh (1972) virtually eradicated late dislocation from their communities. This contrasts with the difficulties of organizing such a service in rural areas. This is reflected in the increased incidence of overlooked dislocations reported from Aberdeen (MacKenzie, 1972) and Northern Ireland (Williamson, 1972).

Lastly there are, as already mentioned, those who have irreducible dislocations at birth characterized by an absence of the clunk sign and a positive abduction in flexion test. There may in addition be another poorly recognized group. From time to time we see a child who has been walking for several months and then suddenly starts to limp. The radiograph discloses a high subluxation verging on dislocation. If the parents are intelligent and observant they will identify the day and time at which this happened and will be confident that all was well previously. Some of these had been examined as babies and presumably no abnormality was found. We may assume primary acetabular dysplasia to be responsible but remain uncertain whether such a condition is identifiable at birth.

The incidence of instability with a positive clunk sign varies greatly in reported series depending upon the enthusiasm of the examiner and the age at which the test is applied. Barlow (1962) reported positive findings in the ratio of 1:67 births; Von Rosen (1968), 1:77, and Small (1968), 1:120 babies examined very soon after birth. The national incidence of true dislocation is about 1.5 per 1 000 live births so it is evident that spontaneous correction is the usual outcome. Mitchell reports that the clunk sign was positive in only 3 per 1 000 births when babies a few days old were examined whereas more than twice this number had been detected by paediatricians immediately after birth. At three weeks Nelson (1966) found the sign positive in 1:290 which approximates very closely to the expected incidence of dislocation at 1.5 per 1 000. These observations will greatly influence our method of management. (*See below*)

Loss of abduction in flexion at birth is probably of greater significance. Wilkinson (1972) found abnormal signs in 37 babies (about 1.1 per 1 000), 23 had a persistent clunk and 14 limited abduction with shortening of whom 6 were detected at birth. Four of the latter group have already undergone operative reduction and acetabular reconstruction is anticipated in a similar number. MacKenzie (1972) also emphasizes the importance of limited abduction. At birth abnormal hips were unstable in 78 per cent and 'stiff' in 22 per cent. At 6 weeks some of both groups had become normal and some unstable hips had become stiff so that the ratio was now 13%:16%.

Limitation of abduction within the first three months is always significant for this sign suggests one of three possibilities. First, it may indicate irreducible dislocation present since birth. Secondly, an unstable reducible hip may have become irreducible. Lastly (and most commonly), it may be due to fixed pelvic obliquity which, as previously indicated, is important on its own account. (*See* p. 46)

Enough has been said to emphasize the problems of organization of efficient neonatal screening and the variability in both the incidence and variety of the signs found and of the outcome. In spite of wide publicity and optimism, can we convince ourselves that screening is indeed a useful contribution? Under ideal circumstances the answer must be 'yes' and it is therefore incumbent upon us to provide such conditions. Some will inevitably escape detection and present themselves later with frank dislocation, but in number they will be well below that expected in unscreened communities being of the order of 1:10 000. There will, in addition, be those mistakenly regarded as stabilized who subsequently prove not to be so. Such children are in an advantageous position for they are likely to be detected at follow-up examination at a stage when secondary changes are minimal and the outcome of either conservative or operative treatment will probably be favourable.

This, however, is not the final word for we must still consider the timing of screening and methods of management in relation to a condition which is generally self-correcting. It is convenient to screen shortly after birth but if administratively possible it might well be preferable to postpone the examination for a month or six weeks. By this age most will be normal and those who are not will display unequivocal signs and active treatment will be clearly indicated. Furthermore, at this age radiographs may be helpful, the parents will have been spared unnecessary anxiety, and most importantly, the hazards of early splinting will be reduced. There is no evidence to suggest that the outcome would be less favourable in those who have persisting signs of either instability or limited abduction.

Splinting in abduction was at one time the immediate reaction when positive signs were detected in the newborn. Further experience, however, has taught us that this is not absolutely necessary and may in fact be harmful. From the evidence of many surveys we know that most babies with hip instability become stable within three weeks, so, at best, wholesale treatment is generally over-treatment. Furthermore, we should not ignore the consequences of causing unwarranted anxiety in the mind of a recently-delivered mother. Of greater importance is the fact that the risk of damaging the epiphyseal nucleus and even the growth plate is not negligible if we apply a splint which enforces constant pressure in the abducted and flexed position (*Figure 2.4*).

A mode of management should take these factors into account and should also distinguish clearly between instability alone, instability with some loss of abduction, and loss of abduction without instability. Simple instability with a positive Barlow sign and full abduction has a generally favourable outcome. Re-examination at about three weeks will confirm that the hip is clinically normal in all but very few. Those who are normal (these include some in whom a positive sign had been reported which was absent on the first hospital examination) need no immediate treatment but it is our practice to examine them again at 4 months and 1 year both clinically and radiologically. These ages are chosen because at 4 months an abnormal radiograph is readily interpretable and at 1 year we may anticipate that walking is imminent and this seems an appropriate time for the final examination. If, on the other hand, instability persists at 3 weeks it would seem logical to treat the hip by splinting in abduction. We believe that the method used should be proof against over-enthusiastic abduction, unauthorized removal by the mother (more commonly the grandmother), and should permit freedom of movement within a prescribed range of safety. Many of the splints in common use do not fulfil these criteria in any respect and for this reason we prefer a miniature Denis Browne Harness (*see* p.62). This is applied without pressure and maintains this position without interruption if the webbing bandoliers are stitched in position. Any interference is readily detected and the child is easily cleaned without removing the splint. There is furthermore a prescribed range of active movement in all directions which enables the older babies to crawl at their appointed time. Such freedom, convenience, and safety encourages the mother to accept the method and she will seldom request that the splint be removed prematurely. The surgeon is therefore under no pressure to cease treatment before walking is due to begin though he will generally be satisfied with the situation after six months. It may be desirable to change the splint twice during this period to allow for growth and because of contamination but this is not always necessary for many of the parts are adjustable and replaceable. Surveillance should continue for several years for sometimes the femoral head stands away from the acetabulum and we must then distinguish between persisting anteversion or intra-articular obstruction (*see* p.63).

When there is limitation of abduction a new and more important component emerges. There is now a very real danger of damaging the epiphysis or growth plate if any force is used in the application of a splint. Fixed pelvic obliquity will be the usual explanation and the management of this will be discussed (p. 46). Of the remainder, most will continue to be associated with a persisting clunk sign but the implication is that irreducibility is imminent. A smaller number, in whom there is no clunk and in whom there is no evidence of pelvic

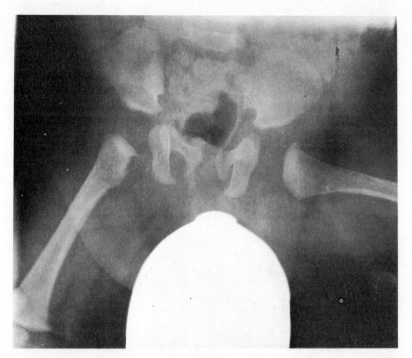

Figure 2.1. (a) The right hip is seen to be abducted

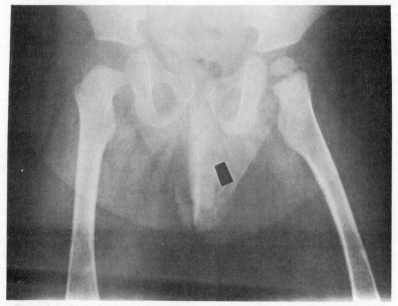

Figure 2.1. (b) 1 year post the application of a pillow splint for 3 months. There is a delay in ossification

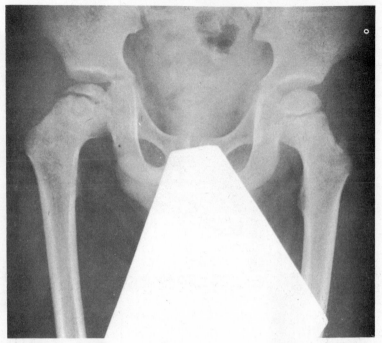

Figure 2.1. (c) The appearance 6 years later. There is persisting damage to the femoral head

obliquity, will be examples of true congenital dislocation. These are detectable in a well centred radiograph both by a displacement and also by the presence of a concavity above the acetabulum with a dense medial wall which suggests that a false acetabulum has already formed. In either event, splinting in the position of deformity, i.e. with uncorrected limitation of abduction, is useless and potentially harmful for it will be natural to attempt to restore abduction by the 'gentle' pressure of a tight splint (*Figure 2.1*).

If limited abduction is associated with persistence of the clunk it is best to perform adductor tenotomy before splinting. Great care must be exercised when the splint is applied under anaesthesia not to secure the hip at the extreme of the range attainable, for in the conscious child this may well amount to undesirable tension. When true congenital dislocation is suspected, reduction must be obtained first for otherwise we will not only be splinting the hip in a position of deformity but also subjecting the femoral head to compression against the pelvic wall and greatly hazarding the blood supply (*Figure 2.2*). These babies should be treated by preliminary traction with adductor tenotomy as though the diagnosis had been made at a later date (*see* page 54). Unfortunately, even at this age, it may not be possible to reduce such a dislocation by non-operative methods and surgical treatment will be indicated later. We must then assume that the dislocation has occurred during intra-uterine life and that secondary changes have already supervened by the time of birth. If reduction fails it is of course essential not to splint the hip in the position of displacement while awaiting operation, for this is useless and likely to be damaging.

In conclusion, we must concede that the results of treatment of established dislocation presenting after walking begins remain a source of dissatisfaction. We will congratulate ourselves frequently during the early years after reduction and demonstrate our handiwork with pride, but as we follow these patients into

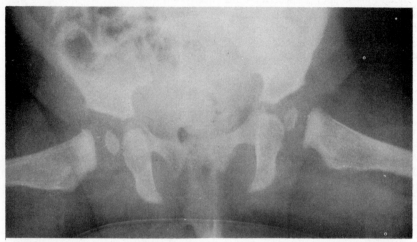

Figure 2.2. (a) At 6 months the plaster has just been removed post 3 months immobilization

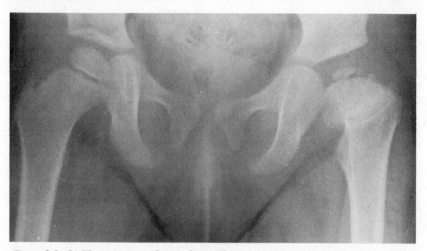

Figure 2.2. (b) The appearance 3 years later. The proximal femur is clearly damaged. The outcome was similar to that illustrated in Figure 2.4. (c)

adolescence and early adult life disquieting symptoms or radiological signs begin to emerge in too many of our apparently successful early results. That we must seek alternative methods by concentrating upon diagnosis within the first few weeks of life is obvious. There are, to be sure, difficulties in organization and potential errors in management possibly resulting in unnecessary damage to hips which might, if untreated, have developed normally. Nonetheless, if the principles are well understood and mistakes avoided we may reasonably expect an improvement in our long-term results as a result of this new philosophy. At the very least there is now a high index of suspicion among medical and lay people which can only be beneficial. We are, of course, still seeing undiagnosed dislocations in spite of screening but there is no doubt that we are seeing them earlier and at a time when secondary changes have not become established as formidable barriers to reduction. The result is that correction is now being achieved by gentler methods of which non-surgical techniques remain the most desirable. If surgery is necessary this is far less radical than we are accustomed to use in neglected patients.

PELVIC OBLIQUITY

Screening of newborn babies to detect instability has led to the increasing recognition of fixed pelvic obliquity in which one hip has restriction of abduction and the other restriction of adduction. The hip with limited abduction will also be apparently short so that the baby presents with signs clinically indistinguishable from those of congenital dislocation. The radiograph excludes dislocation but may be wrongly interpreted as showing acetabular insufficiency. Careful scrutiny, however, will disclose that the pelvis is oblique for the obturator foramina are asymmetrical and the ilium above the allegedly dysplastic acetabulum is narrower than its fellow (*Figure 2.3(a)*). If doubt persists the radiograph should be repeated with the legs abducted as far as possible which will accentuate the apparent differences between the two sides. The distinction between true acetabular dysplasia and this artefact is important for two reasons. Firstly, if adduction is allowed to persist, true secondary acetabular dysplasia and sub-luxation may develop and it is for this reason that we include the syndrome within the spectrum of congenital dislocation. Secondly, if treated in abduction with the use of any force, ischaemic necrosis is a significant hazard (*Figure 2.4(c)*).

Although these patients may be referred during the neonatal period we more commonly see them between three and six months of age. The neonatal presentation however suggests that this is the result of intra-uterine malposition though we cannot exclude the effect of the baby habitually lying on one side in those seen later. There appear to be two varieties. One is part of a general moulding syndrome and is seen together with plagiocephaly, infantile idiopathic scoliosis, postural talipes and rib moulding. The second is a separate entity unassociated with other manifestations.

Pelvic obliquity is commonly seen with infantile scoliosis as a component of the moulded-baby syndrome (Lloyd-Roberts and Pilcher, 1965). The obliquity is simply the result of the scoliosis and it is particularly evident when the baby is viewed in suspension from behind for the pelvis will be seen to follow the curve of the spine so that it is raised on the concave side. The prognosis for infantile idiopathic scoliosis presenting within the first year was very favourable in 92 per cent of our patients and as the scoliosis resolves so the pelvic obliquity diminishes. Indeed, the hip on the concave side caused concern in only one patient. The nature of the moulded-baby syndrome is of some importance in considering the cause of this variety of pelvic obliquity. The moulding mal-formation is acquired for it is not present at birth. It is much less commonly seen today than it was ten years ago. Further retrospective investigation of our patients (Cook and Pilcher, 1977) has shown a significant relationship between this variety of scoliosis and the preferred lying position. Babies with left-sided curves lie on the right side and have pelvic obliquity orientated towards adduction on the right. This type therefore seems to be the result of habitual side-lying and consequent adduction of the lower hip. The present rarity of this pattern of scoliosis is attributable to the adoption of prone-lying as a routine practice. This is longstanding in the United States, where infantile scoliosis is very uncommon. The prognosis for spontaneous resolution without permanent damage to the hip is therefore excellent in this variety for it is due to the cause of the associated scoliosis and governed by its prognosis.

Pelvic obliquity without scoliosis differs in many respects. It is present at birth which implies an abnormal fetal posture, is less likely to resolve rapidly and spontaneously and, if uncorrected, it places the adducted hip at risk to subluxation. The condition may be described as due to fixed pelvic abduction or adduction. Badgley and O'Connor (1953) and Weissman (1954) prefer the former description whereas Lloyd-Roberts and Swann (1966) favour adduction to emphasize the risk to the hip on this side. In either event, the signs are similar, being a relative increase in abduction on one side and restriction on the other. Weissman, however, believes that abduction is the primary fault and is followed later by contralateral adduction. Catterall (1977) has also considered the nature of pelvic obliquity in relation to true acetabular dysplasia. While confirming limitation of abduction he has noted an increase in adduction and flexion and an altered arc of rotation on the same side. If the radiograph is repeated in varying positions of pelvic rotation and obliquity the apparently deficient acetabulum can be shown to be normal in profile as, indeed, one would expect. However a consideration of both the clinical and radiological evidence suggests that the acetabulum may be incorrectly orientated (anteverted) though otherwise normal in contour. If this is confirmed, pelvic obliquity becomes an unquestionable variant on the theme of congenital dislocation.

Whatever the mechanism, its recognition should alert the clinician to the possibility of delayed subluxation. Routine examination of the newborn should include comparison of leg lengths and the range of abduction in flexion both on this account and also to detect prenatal dislocation. The syndrome is probably more common than we think and may be the cause of subluxation in some patients who present later and are categorized as suffering from primary subluxation with acetabular deficiency (*Figure 2.3*).

The prognosis is presented by Weissman in relation to the degree of abduction contracture in one hip and adduction in the other. The abduction contracture always resolved progressively but this was less constant on the adducted side. Of 51 patients adduction ('dysplasia') resolved spontaneously in 13. Of those treated in abduction 26 corrected rapidly and 10 slowly. Dislocation occurred in 2, one of whom had been treated in abduction from birth.

Treatment is less simple than it would seem for splinting in abduction, which is the logical approach, is not always entirely successful for a predisposition to femoral capital ischaemia is a significant complication. In its ultimate form this is seen in patients in whom pelvic obliquity has not been recognized and the hip manipulated on the mistaken diagnosis of dislocation. Severe ischaemia involving the growth plate is almost inevitable resulting in secondary coxa vara, shortening

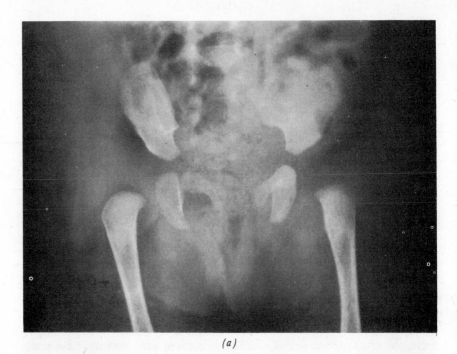

(a)

(b)

Figure 2.3. (a) The appearance is of pelvic obliquity. Note the difference between the ilia. (b) There is still slight obliquity and subluxation is occurring.

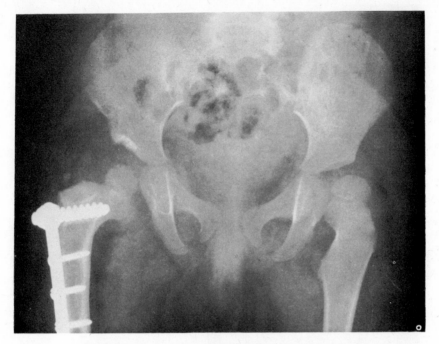

Figure 2.3.(c) An osteotomy was necessary to restore congruity

of the femoral neck and overgrowth of the trochanter (*Figure 2.4*). Although this is an extreme example it serves to emphasize the very real danger of ischaemia if abduction is forced and the hip maintained in this position. Providing that the epiphysis alone is affected, recovery to a spherical head shape is probable but if the growth plate is damaged the consequences may be grave. It has been our practice to teach the mother abduction stretching exercises if the baby presents within the first three months of life. If seen later or the contracture has not yielded we have advised adductor tenotomy and the use of Denis Browne's controlled-movement abduction harness (*see* page 62). This is, in general, a satisfactory method but we must still be wary of using any force in the application of the splint. I suspect that in two patients in whom there was evidence of segmental necrosis we should have used plaster in a position of less abduction.

MANAGEMENT OF CONGENITAL DISLOCATION BEYOND THE NEONATAL PERIOD

Discussion of management divides itself naturally into three sections according to the age at which the child is presented for treatment. Firstly we may consider the infant at less than one year, secondly the child at one to six years and lastly those over six. The age of six is chosen somewhat arbitrarily for the sake of presentation, but clearly there will be some overlap between the methods used for those a year or two older or younger than this.

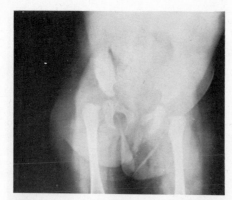

Figure 2.4. (a) There is obliquity of the pelvis

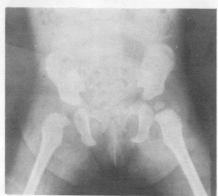

Figure 2.4. (b) Following treatment in abduction, capital ossification is delayed due to ischaemia

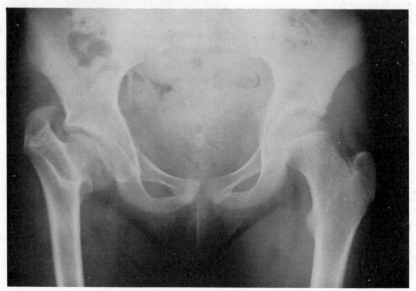

Figure 2.4. (c) There has been premature closure of the capital epiphysis, shortening of the neck and overgrowth of the trochanter

DISLOCATION IN INFANCY

Two different varieties are seen. Firstly, there is the rare irreducible dislocation presenting at the time of neonatal screening. The signs are the same as those of dislocation at any age (limitation of abduction in flexion and shortening in the unilateral) and of pelvic obliquity. The radiograph distinguishes them. Although rare, this may occur more frequently than we think for, obsessed with his efforts to elicit a clunk, the examiner may overlook these signs. These are intra-uterine dislocations and, in spite of early diagnosis, they often respond poorly to conservative treatment so that delay in diagnosis is less damaging than one might suppose (*Figure 2.5*).

The second variety is made up of those unstable hips which do not correct themselves and may result from either failure to recognize instability at the neonatal examination or, if so recognized, from failure to treat persisting instability with sufficient vigour. Delay in diagnosis is often attributable to overconfidence in the reliability of neonatal screening and disregard of the mother's complaints of difficulty in putting on the nappy, asymmetry etc. Unlike the first variety, delay is detrimental for in these cases conservative treatment will usually succeed at this age.

Babies with limited abduction which indicates irreducible dislocation require the full conservative regime of traction, tenotomy, plaster and harness – to be described later – regardless of age. We, too often, see failure attributable to the belief that the very young need no more than splinting in abduction. This at best does no greater harm than postponing the start of proper treatment, but at worst it causes epiphyseal and growth-plate ischaemia or damage to the articular surface of the femoral head if any force is used in applying the splint.

If traction fails to reduce the hip and operation is to be performed later, it is essential that the temptation to splint the hip in abduction during the waiting period be resisted. It is better to allow freedom from restraint expecting that increased mobility and muscular development will be encouraged by crawling. It is certainly always useless and often harmful to splint the hip in the dislocated position.

There are differences of opinion about the timing and technique of operation during the first year of life. Some surgeons proceed to immediate open reduction by the conventional anterior approach, others prefer the perineal operation (Mau *et al.*, 1971) at this age, and still others postpone operation until the child is one year of age.

The perineal approach is gaining in popularity especially on the continent of Europe and its proponents argue that its simplicity, safety and effectiveness make it the method of choice at any time within the first year. My personal experience is limited to a very few patients operated upon more than 10 years ago. The operation is certainly simple and enables the surgeon to release both tight adductors and iliopsoas for their own sake and to improve access. A good view of the floor of the acetabulum is obtained and any obstruction readily removed. The quality of reduction obtained did not, however, satisfy me, but this may have been due to inexperience with the technique or because of my inability to reach an inverted labrum in the roof. Other disadvantages are that the siting of the wound is in an inevitably contaminated area and damage to the blood supply to the femoral epiphysis which will be considered further. Although

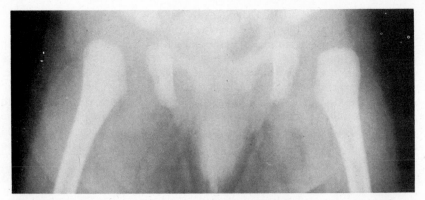

Figure 2.5. (a) Within days of birth there was a clunk on the right. On the left there was no clunk but abduction was limited. Note the similarity between the appearances

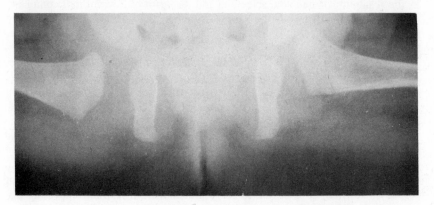

Figure 2.5. (b) Following traction the left hip failed to reduce

this method is less favoured in this country than elsewhere, we should for the moment keep an open mind on it and study the long-term results as they emerge.

The crux of the issue concerns the relative risk of epiphyseal ischaemia. Using the perineal approach, I twice divided a vessel lying on the inferior surface of the joint capsule which seemed to be an important contributor to the epiphyseal circulation. Branches of the circumflex femoral arteries are frequently divided in the approach but advocates of the method assert that this has no adverse effect. It may in fact be that the vessels entering the head which arise from the metaphysis and cross the growth plate provide an adequate collateral supply. This arrangement is peculiar to the age of infancy (Trueta, 1957) but does not, however, seem to compensate as effectively when the anterior approach is used at this age. Several surgeons independently have noted an increased incidence of ischaemia when open reduction is performed at this age in this manner (Lloyd-Roberts and Swann, 1966; Trevor, personal communication). They consequently prefer to delay their intervention until the child is about one year of age by which time this risk appears to be diminished. This remains their practice for this reason alone since there is no special technical difficulty nor,

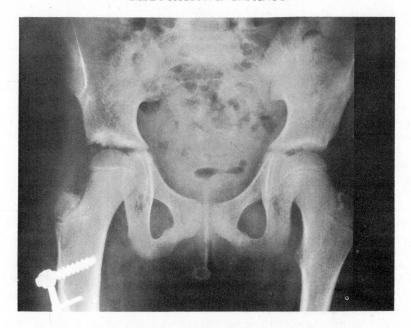

Figure 2.5. (c) Open reduction and osteotomy was necessary later

today, any undue anaesthetic hazard peculiar to this age. It would, otherwise, seem preferable to operate as soon as the indication was plain on the principle that the sooner the dislocation is corrected the more normal the development of the hip is likely to be.

It is perhaps surprising that so many of these very young children require open reduction especially when neonatal screening is a routine practice. The explanation, probably, is that true intra-uterine dislocations are often detected at this age and these cannot, in general, be satisfactorily reduced by gentle, non-operative means. These dislocations tend to be 'tight' which implies that the femoral head is closely apposed to the pelvic wall, so that it is not uncommon to notice a false acetabulum on the radiograph and at operation before walking begins. This suggests that dislocation has been present for longer than we think, including a variable proportion of the stage of fetal growth. It is not surprising, therefore, that soft tissues are contracted and resistant to stretching and that the acetabulum, lacking the stimulation of a contained head, develops poorly. It is among this group that we meet some of our most difficult cases. In contrast, most of the unstable hips which become dislocated respond well to non-operative treatment because dislocation occurs later, so that soft tissue contracture is acquired rather than congenital and the acetabulum has been stimulated. Further-more, joint laxity is common and associated with 'loose' dislocations. Some, however, have persisting acetabular obstruction, usually the inturned labrum (limbus), which requires removal. Not all the others develop normally so that innominate or femoral osteotomy may be indicated later.

DISLOCATION BETWEEN ONE AND SIX YEARS

The age of six is chosen because this is the time when we must seriously consider the wisdom of treating bilateral dislocations.

General observations

There are three fundamental stages of treatment and one essential principle which applies at all stages. The first stage requires that we achieve congruous reduction as early and as gently as possible and restrict the time of complete immobilization to the minimum. In the second, we must ensure that congruous reduction (which is at first usually in abduction and internal rotation) is equally satisfactory in the erect weight-bearing position. In the third stage, this weight-bearing congruity must be maintained throughout growth during which the hip joint is undergoing continuing change, i.e. normal development modified by the adjustments necessary to correct the secondary effects of dislocation.

The essential principle is to avoid procrastination at all stages and all ages. There is no acceptable compromise between a satisfactory and unsatisfactory situation. If the position at any stage is not good it is bad and demands immediate action to correct the matter.

These are of course desirable generalizations which are applicable in ideal circumstances but not always easily applied, especially when the older child is presented. Some of the problems will be considered later but it is important to appreciate the effect of age of reduction upon the subsequent development of the hip. Bilateral dislocation is also an adverse factor when each hip is considered separately.

Age affects the chances of success of each stage. Increasing age and bilaterality both combine to prevent satisfactory non-operative reductions in the first stage, so that the operation rate rises until, beyond the age of two years, it becomes the rule rather than the exception. Secondly, they also predispose to greater secondary structural changes, and increase the operative indications to stabilize reduction in the erect position. Thirdly, an inadequate acetabular response to the delayed normal stimulus frequently indicates a secondary operation during further growth.

Finally, even if the dislocation is unilateral, the opposite hip may well be dysplastic or subluxated and must be treated with equal vigour. It will be an advantage in the future to have one normal hip if the result on the dislocated side is less satisfactory than we might wish.

Conservative treatment

(a) *Reduction*

Although an entirely non-operative regime is only likely to succeed when the child is under two years of age, affected on only one side and loose jointed, the importance of this approach cannot be overemphasized for three reasons. Firstly, our best results are obtained when we can avoid operation, providing that no mistakes are made and no surgical indication ignored. Secondly, non-operative reduction reduces the severity of any subsequent operation to one of stabilization alone with consequent improvement in the outcome. Thirdly, even if unsuccessful, preliminary traction simplifies a late open reduction by stretching soft tissues and thereby reduces the severity of the operation and the degree of anatomical rearrangement, thus favouring the integrity of the vascular supply.

Primary manipulation followed by immobilization in 90° of abduction and flexion (or even more flexion) is, or should be, obsolete. The incidence of both imperfect reduction and epiphyseal ischaemia is unacceptably high at about 40 per cent (Wilkinson and Carter, 1960). This is not surprising for the frog

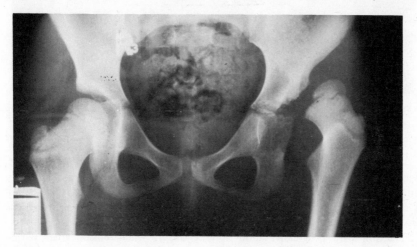

Figure 2.6. (a) Unilateral dislocation of left hip

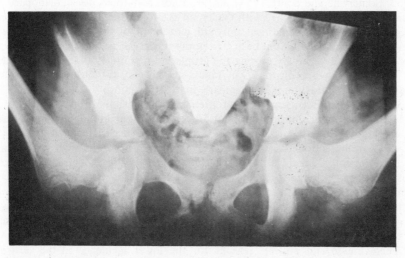

Figure 2.6. (b) To show the position in which the hips were immobilized following manipulative reduction. Both capital epiphyses are dense due to ischaemia

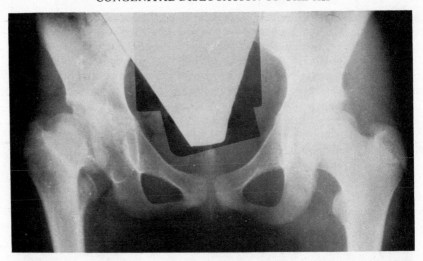

Figure 2.6 (c) Later the right hip which was originally normal is the more severely damaged

position, even without excessive flexion, may cause ischaemia in a normally situated epiphysis (*Figure 2.6*). Salter has rightly observed that the frog position is only appropriate to frogs and advocates the 'human' position in which the hip is immobilized in about 30° less flexion and abduction.

Traction with progressive abduction, tenotomy when tension arises within the adductors, and, finally, cross-traction of some 2 lb applied at a right-angle to the abducted thigh, is now accepted as the proper primary method (Scott, 1953; Somerville and Scott, 1957). These authors and others use an orthopaedic frame, traction being applied with the legs in extension and increasing abduction being obtained by symmetrical outward movement of the leg splints. Some, however, prefer that traction be at first in the vertical plane and that progressive abduction be obtained by moving the unsplinted legs outward and downwards by means of a hoop (*Figure 2.7*). Adductor tenotomy is indicated by tension therein and cross-traction is used similarly in both methods.

Our preference is vertical traction for reasons other than the primary concentric reduction rate, which in both is about 50 per cent for children under two years of age (Lloyd-Roberts and Swann, 1966). The incidence of ischaemia is lower when vertical traction is used but not eliminated entirely, although in 50 consecutive patients studied for this purpose in both the early stages and later (when positive evidence is more readily detectable) there were none with ischaemia. Reported series of frame reduction average 10 per cent but the diagnosis of ischaemia is often somewhat subjective and depends upon the age at review. For example, delay in ossification of the epiphysis may be due to joint dysplasia or ischaemia, and only examination at a later date will resolve the uncertainty.

There are several possible reasons for the lower incidence in the vertical traction method. The hip is at first flexed at 90° thus relaxing the psoas and placing the femoral head behind the acetabulum so that the pull is towards the acetabulum. By contrast, in the horizontal position the head lies above the acetabulum and the pull is opposed by the shortened psoas; greater pressure may therefore be imposed on the head when abduction begins. The legs and pelvis are free of restraint when suspended so that if tension, which hazards the vascular supply, develops on either side the child adjusts the plane of the pelvis to reduce it. This is not possible on the frame, for pelvis and legs are restrained and their relationship enforced by the degree of abduction imposed.

Further advantages of vertical traction are ease of nursing in suspension (comparable to Gallows traction) and its possible application to any cot. The only special requirement is plumber's piping drilled at intervals for the traction cords. In contrast, the frame requires those special nursing skills verging on a mystique usually found in orthopaedic hospitals alone. We have not encountered the vascular accidents to the limb which have been reported when Gallows traction is used for fractures in older children and are confident enough to use it up to four years of age (*Figure 2.7*).

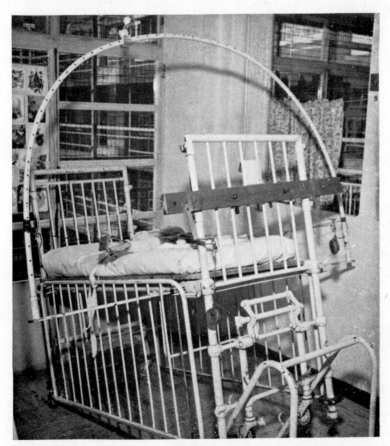

Figure 2.7. (a) Traction using a hoop on an ordinary cot. (Reproduced from Lloyd-Roberts, *Orthopaedics in Infancy and Childhood*, 1971, Butterworths, by permission)

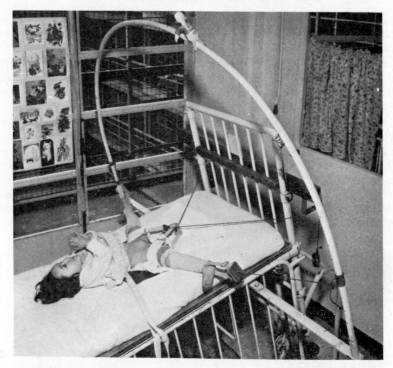

Figure 2.7. (b) Treatment is complete. The legs are fully abducted and cross-traction is being applied. (Reproduced from Lloyd-Roberts, *Orthopaedics in Infancy and Childhood,* 1971, Butterworths, by permission)

Vertical traction without abduction is maintained for 4 days and full abduction achieved about two weeks later. Cross-traction is then applied for 1 week. Tenotomy is usually performed at between 1 week and 10 days. There is no virtue in persisting for more than 4 weeks for there is little prospect of late reduction and stiffness, porosis and even epiphyseal arrest may occur (MacKenzie, Seddon and Trevor, 1960; Borring and Scrase, 1965). Successful reduction is often heralded by an abrupt change in the demeanour of the child. Poised on the brink, she is fretful but she becomes contented suddenly when reduction is complete.

When reviewed after three and four weeks the radiograph discloses one of three situations. Firstly the hip remains dislocated, secondly the epiphysis lies opposite but displaced laterally from the acetabulum, and lastly it is concentrically reduced.

If dislocated we have two alternatives. We may either explore the hip or attempt a gentle manipulative reduction. Once the hip is fully abducted there is little risk of vascular compromise if gentleness is used and a high proportion of them will be felt to reduce. If, however, any obstruction remains within the acetabulum there will be compression between this and the head which may cause deformity later. It may be shown by arthrography that an inverted labrum will yield to the pressure of the head and become flattened against the acetabular roof (Severin, 1950). This compression is undesirable and therefore many, myself included, prefer to proceed to immediate open reduction (Somerville and Scott, 1957) (*Figure 2.8*).

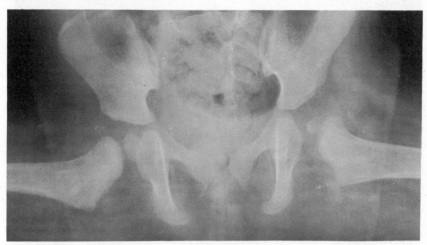

Figure 2.8. (a) The hip on traction is laying away from the acetabulum

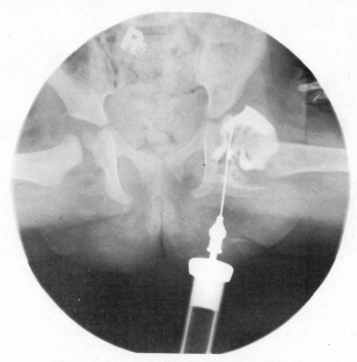

Figure 2.8. (b) An arthrogram reveals an inturned labrum

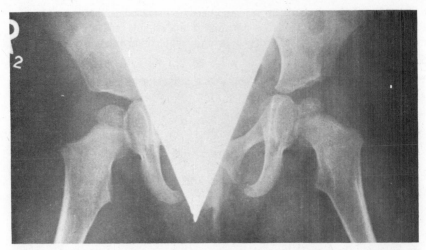

Figure 2.8. (c) On continuing conservative treatment, congruous reduction is obtained but the head has become irregular

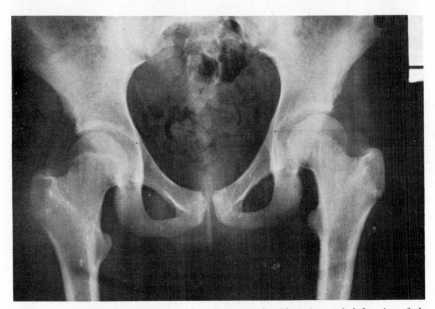

Figure 2.8. (d) 12 years later there is slight upward subluxation and deformity of the femoral head which is poorly covered

The second alternative is lateral without upward displacement. This is not necessarily due to persisting obstruction, for traction in abduction may be the cause especially when there is generalized joint laxity. Additional factors are redundancy of the capsule, or eccentric epiphyseal ossification and anteversion especially if the leg is externally rotated (*Figure 2.9*). If the hip is in fact reduced,

60

a trial period of six weeks in plaster will overcome the effects of traction and laxity and the hip will be satisfactory in the subsequent radiograph. It is undesirable, however, to use plaster for even so short a period if the hip is not reduced, and it is therefore important to distinguish between acceptable and unacceptable lateral displacement. Arthrography will certainly resolve the issue but we may

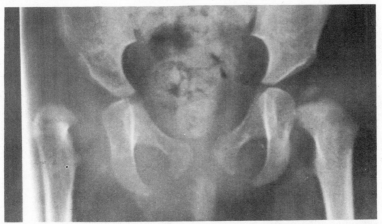

Figure 2.9. (a) The right hip is dislocated, the left is within normal limits

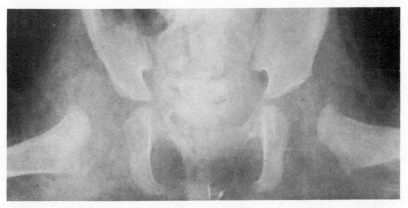

Figure 2.9. (b) After 3 weeks traction, both hips are equally distracted laterally

often decide by examining the hip under anaesthesia whether to proceed to operation or plaster immobilization as indicated by the findings. If examination reveals a hip which in abduction readily dislocates on pressure from before backwards, open reduction follows. Anterior dislocation can also be deceiving if clinical examination with or without anaesthesia is omitted and reliance is placed on the radiograph alone. Overlap may mislead the surgeon into believing that reduction is almost perfect, whereas in fact an obstruction has prevented this and the femoral head has simply moved forward above the acetabulum to lie in front.

(b) *Maintenance and stabilization of reduction*

Having achieved concentric reduction in full abduction, this is usually maintained by plaster in a position less potentially harmful than that of a frog. If the quality of reduction is suspect, special care will be taken at the first plaster change to ensure that the relationship is by now concentric. We may now continue with

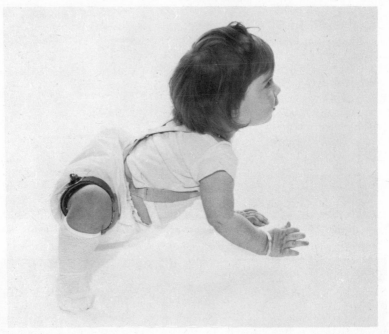

Figure 2.10. To illustrate the Denis Browne controlled-movement hip splint which also allows walking after a fashion

plaster treatment, perhaps, gradually reducing the degree of abduction and flexion and increasing internal rotation, for as we adduct so the significance of anteversion increases.

More recently, however, we have come to recognize the evils of prolonged immobilization – porosis, muscle-wasting, impaired cartilaginous nutrition etc. – and, in the child with a dislocated hip, a lack of that necessary functional activity which stimulates acetabular growth and the undesirable psychological effects of a static life. Furthermore, we now know that concentric reduction is not imperilled provided that we restrict adduction and extension. Consequently controlled-movement splints have evolved such as the Pavlik and Denis Browne harness. Both of these allow movement within the prescribed range and in the second type crawling and walking are possible. The adverse effects are thereby reduced and, furthermore, soiling can be prevented. The hip is available for clinical examination and the radiograph is not obscured by plaster. Should reduction be insecure, redislocation is certain and readily detected so that no time is lost in recognizing the need to operate and the damage that follows immobilization in an eccentric position can be avoided (*Figure 2.10*).

The harness is retained until development of the acetabulum is judged to be adequate — a somewhat vague assertion — but unavoidable, for its important lateral lip is predominantly cartilaginous in early childhood. Arthrography will clarify uncertainty but, in practice, it is usually unnecessary. The time spent in the harness ranges from 6 to 18 months depending upon the age of the child and the degree of dysplasia and this is sometimes extended by using the device as a night splint.

It is our impression that controlled-movement splinting is greatly superior to rigid immobilization in respect of both the quality of hip development and the time taken to achieve this. Comparable series are at present under review (Harris, Catterall and Lloyd-Roberts, 1976).

When the harness is removed and any residual splint stiffness overcome, most patients will be found to maintain congruous reduction when the legs are in the neutral walking position. Some, however, seem laterally displaced from the acetabulum with or without subluxation. Any upward subluxation is an indication for stabilization of the reduction by either re-alignment of the acetabulum (innominate osteotomy) or of the femur by varus rotation osteotomy, for congruous reduction is already possible in abduction. These operations will be discussed later. Lateral displacement may be due to persisting obstruction but this should be very rare for it implies that an error has been made earlier on. Persisting anteversion is the common cause and it may be distinguished from obstruction by arthrography or by a radiograph in the neutral position with internal rotation which restores congruity if anteversion alone is responsible.

An obstruction must be removed by operation but the management of anteversion is more difficult, for it may resolve spontaneously when walking begins. Children under two years of age (or thereabouts) may not have walked, or done so but briefly, before treatment began. In these we may wait for up to a year for derotation to occur, providing that we are vigilant in detecting the onset of upward subluxation. If anteversion still persists or the child has already walked before diagnosis, it is better to correct it by varus derotation osteotomy of the femur.

Lastly, we must ensure that congruity in the position of walking is maintained throughout growth for in some the acetabulum will fail to develop and in others anteversion may recur. Either event will indicate the operation appropriate to the cause of lost congruity.

Operative treatment

The indication is failure to obtain reduction by non-operative means and the incidence is related directly to age. In practice most children over two years of age require operation and in very few children over three years of age is operation avoidable. As in conservative treatment, we must reduce the dislocation, stabilize reduction and maintain congruity till the end of growth.

(a) Open reduction

The operation may be simple or very difficult. A child between one and two years of age who has joint laxity and a unilateral dislocation may require no more than removal of the inturned labrum, followed by a stabilizing operation. In contrast, the older child who has been walking for perhaps 3 years with high bilateral dislocations which are 'tight', i.e. with limited movement in abduction and head closely applied to the pelvic wall, presents technical problems of considerable complexity. The reason for the contrast is shortening of some soft tissues, capsular constriction, and secondary or persisting skeletal anomalies of which anteversion of the acetabulum is the most significant.

In either event our objective must be to obtain congruous and stable reduction without tension. At the end of the operation it should be possible to reduce the hip gently to a depth at which the cartilaginous femoral head completely disappears from view when the leg is abducted and internally rotated. Stability should permit forceful upward pressure in full internal rotation in neutral abduction without redislocation.

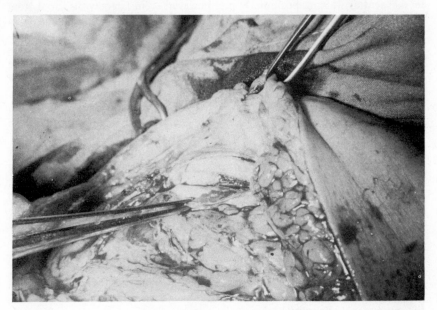

Figure 2.11. Splitting the iliac apophysis

The surgeon must be prepared to vary the extent of his operation in relation to the degree of abnormality present and be prepared to perform those additional steps such as innominate osteotomy or femoral shortening which are sometimes indicated at the time of the first operation. The inexperienced should be strongly advised to begin with the young, the lax and the unilateral, before attempting the more difficult varieties, for the first operation is all-important. Redislocation after operation followed by a further open reduction (possibly repeated) is almost inevitably the forerunner of a less than satisfactory outcome.

Some aspects of the surgical technique merit emphasis. A good general account of open reduction has been written by Scaglietti and Calandriello (1962) and Salter (1967) has described the essential first step of his combined operation to reduce and stabilize the hip. The skin incision is of moment for most are girls and the anterior Smith-Petersen approach leaved an unnecessary blemish. It is better to use a transverse incision in the line of the skin crease from mid-inguinal point to tip of trochanter passing one finger's breadth distal to the anterior superior iliac spine. In closure, the skin edges fall naturally together and may be best secured by subcutaneous and continuous subcuticular suture. The approach is now developed between sartorius and the tensor fascia distally and proximally by bisecting the iliac epiphysis in the sagittal plane so that the lateral half may be stripped outwards in continuity with the periosteum of the wing of the ilium (*Figure 2.11*). Sutures placed between the displaced and attached halves of the apophysis give secure fixation to gluteus medius at the end of the operation. Pelvic deformity due to growth disturbance does not occur when only one half of the apophysis is displaced but may occur if both are so treated when innominate osteotomy is contemplated. Time spent in clearing the capsule of adherent glutei, and the lateral origin of rectus femoris with its overlying fat pad and adherence of capsule to the iliac wing, is well spent. The surgeon should see clearly the front of the capsule from trochanteric line to pelvis especially in its inferior and medial zone. The psoas tendon, being the main upward tether, should always be divided. This may sometimes be difficult unless the leg is abducted and externally rotated, when it may be exposed by splitting the overlying iliacus, rolling the subjacent psoas medially and inspecting the surface which crosses the pubic ramus. Care should be taken to ensure that the whole tendon is divided. The less experienced will be reassured if the femoral nerve is seen. The capsule may now be opened and the method of doing this is important, for in ensuring access we must not compromise stability in internal rotation nor the capacity to reef the capsule later as a check ligament to external rotation. An incision parallel to and half a centimetre from the rim of the acetabulum begins just behind the highest point and continues distally and medially as far as possible. A second incision runs from the starting point towards the great trochanter so that an inverted 'V' is fashioned. This, while giving good access, preserves the posterior capsule as a barrier against which the head may be internally rotated and in repair internal rotation may be stabilized if excess capsule is excised from the apex of the 'V'. This gives a linear suture line to the capsule still attached to the acetabular rim and the inferior iliac spine. This is Salter's method which is always desirable in order to reduce the risk of redislocation anteriorly and is essential if innominate osteotomy is to be performed to prevent posterior dislocation when the hip is internally rotated.

If the ligamentum teres is intact it will lead to the floor of the acetabulum. When it is detached from the head there is no bleeding but this may be brisk proximally from beneath the transverse ligament. This, however, is easily controlled by pressure. The acetabulum is now cleared of its contents so that finally both the cartilaginous and bony components are clearly seen. This involves excision of the labrum (limbus), ligamentum teres and fat pad. In high dislocations a fold of inferior capsule will bulge over the transverse ligament into the joint and both should be divided.

Lastly, it may sometimes be difficult to find the acetabulum especially when there is no ligamentum teres and the inferior capsule is folded upwards to cover the entrance and forms with the superior capsule a narrow isthmus which still further obscures the situation. The isthmus should have been opened by the first capsular incision and access so established, but if this has not been done the

65

incision should now be modified to achieve this. A seeker will identify the floor and clearance can proceed above and below this point. Sometimes acetabular anteversion is such that it lies in front of the anterior inferior spine and is completely covered by capsule. Remembering this, the surgeon will search much further forward and lower than he expects and will resist the temptation to declare the acetabulum absent.

We are now in a position to apply the tests of adequate reduction in respect of both depth and stability as previously described. If these are satisfactory, closure, using the steps already mentioned, is followed by plaster in full internal rotation, some 40° of abduction and 20° of flexion, with the knee flexed to relax the hamstrings. The stabilizing operation will be considered later.

Let us now consider the problem posed when reduction fails to meet the criteria of acceptability. These are: insufficient depth of reduction, tension and persisting instability on upward pressure in internal rotation. Insufficient depth is occasionally due to a normal head poorly contained by an inadequate acetabulum so that one has the impression that the head is too big for the socket. More commonly, some obstruction persists which is usually caused by either failure to remove the whole limbus or by capsule overlying the transverse ligament. Too much tension may be caused by recurrence of adductor contracture as the hip comes down, incomplete division of the psoas, or inadequate release of the glutei from the iliac crest. If tension persists after attention to these, the knee should be flexed to relax the hamstrings. If tension is relieved the first plaster is applied in this position. If tension is not overcome we must shorten the femur. Inadequate depth of reduction or instability which are not corrected by these manoeuvres indicate operations to deepen or re-align the acetabulum. These, together with femoral shortening, will be considered later.

(b) *Stabilizing reduction in the erect position*

This is the next essential step. It is possible to establish this by non-operative means in some patients. Open reduction is regarded as the equivalent of closed reduction and we proceed similarly. However it is generally better to stabilize by operation, for prolonged limitation of movement after open reduction may be followed by troublesome stiffness and this delays the start of normal walking which is the main stimulus to hip joint development.

Having achieved congruous reduction in abduction and internal rotation it is necessary to change the orientation of either the acetabulum or the femur or sometimes both to enable this congruity to be maintained in the position of walking. Although there is debate about the relative merits of acetabular re-alignment ('Innominate osteotomy' − Salter) and the femoral, it must be appreciated that the principle underlying both is the same. Innominate osteotomy re-aligns the anteverted anteriorly-deficient acetabulum with the anteverted and valgus femoral neck, whereas femoral osteotomy re-aligns in the opposite direction. If congruity is restored and maintained by either method, subsequent development of the untreated component will usually be satisfactory. Thus, following innominate osteotomy, femoral valgus and anteversion will decrease and, after femoral osteotomy, satisfactory acetabular development may be confidently anticipated up to the age of four years (Harris, Lloyd-Roberts and Gallien, 1975) (*Figure 2.12*) (Table 2.I) (Sallis and Smith, 1965) (Table 2.II).

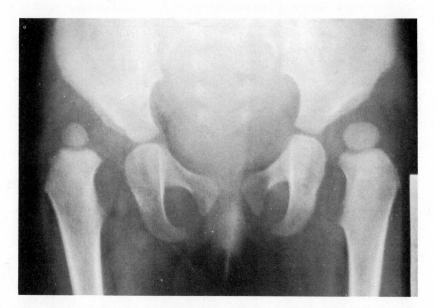

Figure 2.12. (a) Unilateral dislocation on the left with contralateral subluxation at the age of 3½ years

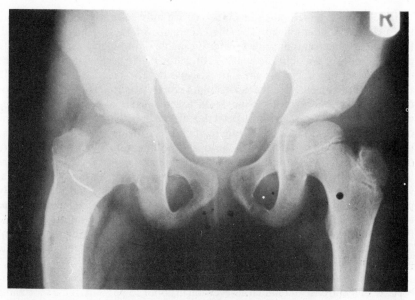

Figure 2.12. (b) At 8 years, following open reduction and femoral osteotomy, acetabular development is satisfactory

TABLE 2.1
Acetabular development related to congruity and the age at which it is obtained

Category	Number of hips	Congruity throughout	Average age of congruity (months)	Late congruity over 3 years	Average age of late congruity (months)	Congruity lost. Not corrected	Never congruous
Normal	53	53	37	18	52	0	0
Good	15	9	48	10	55	5	1
Fair	8	2	36	5	54	3	3
Poor	9	2	45	4	52	3	4
All hips	85	66	41.5	37	53	11	8

TABLE 2.II
Relationship between original cartilage and acetabular angles and final acetabular angle in normal and abnormal hips (*see page 82*)

Final acetabular angle	Cases	
	Normal hips	Abnormal hips
Greater (worse) than initial acetabular angle	1	2
Equal to initial acetabular angle	–	1
Between initial cartilage angle and acetabular angle	7	22
Equal to initial cartilage angle	–	7
Less (better) than initial cartilage angle	–	10

In selecting the method to be employed we must take into account not only the anatomical situation but also the experience of the surgeon in this field. Innominate osteotomy in skilled hands is capable of producing results which are probably unsurpassed, but the penalties of failure due to neglect of those minutiae of technique which are essential to success are grievous. Two examples will suffice. Re-alignment of the acetabulum corrects anteversion and anterior deficiency admirably but by the same token creates a posterior deficiency exposing the head to the risk of posterior dislocation. This is preventable if the capsular repair is assiduous. Secondly, failure to divide the psoas may cause undesirable compression between head and acetabulum. Furthermore, failure of this operation due to technical error may present almost insoluble problems to the surgeon called upon to operate the second time. In contrast, femoral varus osteotomy and external rotation osteotomy are simple and if incorrectly performed may be repeated without undue difficulty. The technique is similar to that used in Perthes' disease (*see* page 137) and should be intertrochanteric for thereby the lesser trochanter is rotated forwards so augmenting the power of iliopsoas as an internal rotator. Moreover, the varus component reduces the pressure between head and acetabulum.

The major disadvantages of femoral osteotomy are the need to repeat it because of recurrence of femoral anteversion in about 15 per cent, some shortening due to the varus element, and the necessity to perform two operations. Femoral stabilization is performed about six weeks after open reduction, whereas the innominate is usually concurrent with open reduction. Sometimes, however, obstinate femoral deformity will indicate this osteotomy to support the stability of an innominate re-alignment.

Protagonists of either can argue in favour of the use of their preference in almost all circumstances, but we may now consider how a surgeon familiar with both methods might apply them discerningly. Femoral osteotomy, as mentioned elsewhere, has a particular appeal when open reduction is unnecessary, i.e. for some patients with reducible subluxations and for some following congruous reduction by conservative methods (*see* page 63). When open reduction is necessary, the test of stability positive, and the child under four years of age, both methods are equally applicable. If the child is over four years of age or the hip is unstable on testing, the innominate osteotomy is clearly indicated as it certainly is when subluxation is associated with acetabular deficiency (*see* page 88). There must remain, however, a sense of disquiet when innominate osteotomy is performed for children over the age of four. Between 1½ and 4 years of age 93 per cent obtained good results but these fall to 56 per cent between the ages of 4 and 16 years (Salter, 1967). Comparable figures are not available for femoral osteotomy but we have shown that acetabular development is unlikely to be satisfactory if congruity is not obtained before the age of four. Thus the results of femoral osteotomy are probably no better and some form of acetabular operation will be needed. Some degree of ischaemia is certainly more common in the older children whatever the method employed. This had prompted some surgeons to advise that the acetabular operation be performed at some time after open reduction so returning again to a two-stage procedure.

Innominate osteotomy in skilled hands is, however, applicable not only when it is specifically indicated, but also as an alternative to femoral osteotomy in other situations, though it may sometimes be necessary to use both. In most, however, reduction and stabilization are achieved safely in one operation if innominate osteotomy is used, whereas it is undesirable to combine femoral osteotomy with open reduction unless concurrent femoral shortening is necessary (*see* page 73) for stability because the vascular supply may be compromised thereby.

When acetabular reconstruction is clearly indicated, an alternative is to deepen the roof of the acetabulum by a turn-down acetabuloplasty supported by a graft. This operation does not re-align the acetabulum but merely deepens it so that re-alignment must be achieved at femoral level. The results are inferior to those of innominate osteotomy when used at the time of open reduction, success being 73 per cent overall compared with 93 per cent success with innominate osteotomies with children under four years of age, but when children are over four years of age the difference is less marked (Trevor, Johns and Fixsen, 1975).

Two further methods of acetabular re-alignment merit attention. Firstly, triple osteotomy (Steele, 1973) in which ilium, ischium and pubis are divided to obtain more acetabular displacement than is possible with ilium alone. The operation is more formidable and although I have no personal experience of it the notion is attractive and the early results encouraging. We must await later results in more patients. Secondly, the acetabular cartilage may be detached from its bed with a thin layer of bone and re-aligned. This is less attractive in concept and outcome because of the risk of chondrolysis.

The principle of stabilization of reduction in the erect position remains valid but the method by which this should be achieved remains uncertain, particularly in the older child. In those less than four years of age, however, innominate and femoral osteotomies are probably comparable in outcome when used during primary treatment (Somerville, 1967). Differences in average age at diagnosis, differences in length of follow-up and in methods of assessment between series permit no greater conviction than this.

(c) *Maintenance of congruous reduction in the erect position*

During continuing growth, incongruity may develop either because of inadequate acetabular growth, recurrence of femoral valgus and anteversion or a combination of both. We have shown that failure to maintain congruity is the commonest cause of acetabular maldevelopment so we must be constantly on the alert (Harris, Lloyd-Roberts and Gallien, 1975) (Table 2.I).

The first essential is to maintain radiological supervision until the end of growth and to act immediately when congruity is deteriorating. This is easier said than done for the child is likely to be fully active and symptom-free but we must never forget that disabling degenerative changes are probable in early adult life if secondary subluxation is allowed to remain uncorrected.

A minor breech in Shenton's line restored by placing the leg in abduction and internal rotation is an absolute indication for femoral varus rotation osteotomy (*Figure 2.13*). Even minor subluxation may contra-indicate innominate osteotomy alone. Although the femoral head is well covered thereby, it remains laterally displaced and movement is then eccentric. This eccentric movement in the

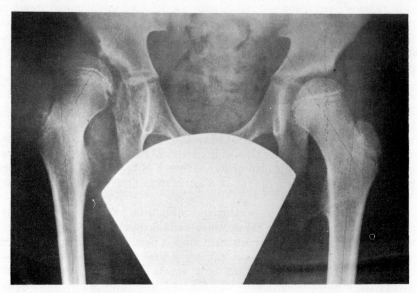

Figure 2.13. (a) At 8 years the left hip is slightly subluxated but the acetabular roof is fair. On the right there is severe subluxation and acetabular deficiency

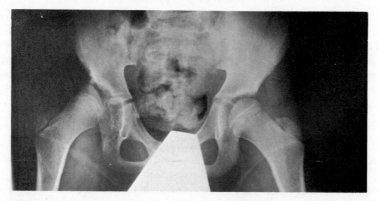

Figure 2.13. (b) Radiograph in abduction and internal rotation restore congruity on the left but the right remains displaced

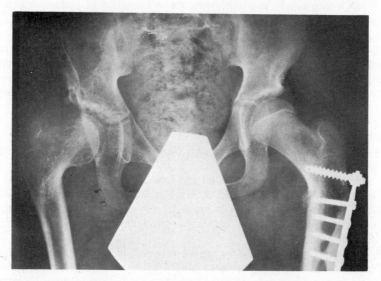

Figure 2.13. (c) 5 years later. Following osteotomy above the left is now satisfactory. The right is greatly improved after open reduction, osteotomy and acetabuloplasty

antero-posterior plane has been emphasized by Somerville (1974) and he implies that a lax anterior capsule and the psoas (now reconstituted) are important factors, for with subluxation the psoas becomes an external rotator pulling the head forwards. Should innominate osteotomy be preferred it will be desirable to reef the capsule and divide the psoas again and even then femoral osteotomy may be needed later. Femoral varus rotation osteotomy protects the head from forward subluxation by positioning it posteriorly and converting the pull of psoas from external to internal rotation. On the other hand, when there is no subluxation but failure of acetabular development (a much less common finding), innominate osteotomy or acetabuloplasty with femoral osteotomy will be appropriate.

If subluxation cannot be reduced by suitable positioning of the leg there has been procrastination and the outlook is compromised for neither stabilizing operation will succeed in the presence of fixed subluxation. It is now necessary to start again with an open reduction before stabilization or to accept the displacement and salvage the situation so far as possible by pelvic osteotomy (Chiari), high-shelf or Colonna arthroplasty (*see* page 74).

MANAGEMENT OVER THE AGE OF SIX

At this age we must consider the advisability of treating children with bilateral dislocations presenting for the first time and accept that virtually all hips will require acetabular re-alignment or reconstruction.

When dislocations are bilateral and the child's function is good, great care must be taken in selection, for operation may now be a surgical adventure of little benefit to the patient. There are two contrasting patterns. In the first the child has a surprisingly good gait with severe limitation of abduction and well formed false acetabulae with which the heads articulate (tight dislocations). Although the gait will deteriorate as height and weight increase and early degenerative arthritis is common these are, in general, unsuitable for treatment unless it is understood that loss of function due to stiffness is probable and acceptable as a preliminary to total replacement in later life. Alternatively, the child has a severe limp, joint laxity with a surprising range of abduction and a hip which telescopes freely. The radiograph shows the head lying well away from the iliac wing and no obvious false acetabulum. These children are likely to benefit from operation up to about nine years of age.

Social and racial considerations sometimes influence our decision. Marriage prospects may be prejudiced by a limp or enhanced by the width of the pelvis. The ability to squat may be essential and loss of existing abduction a handicap. Some races respond less well than others. For example, in some Arab countries 4 years is regarded as the upper limit and my experience confirms this, for stiffness and ischaemia seem commoner there than in European or central Mediterranean races.

When one hip is dislocated we are on safer ground. Decision is dominated by the fact that later total replacement cannot be expected to have a satisfactory outcome in untreated dislocations. Furthermore, the limp is unsightly and any postoperative stiffness will be compensated for by the other hip. Mild maldevelopment of the opposite hip is, if anything, an encouragement to proceed for both may benefit from replacement in the future. The radiograph will reveal the favourable or unfavourable features of a 'loose' or 'tight' dislocation to which may be added thickening of the acetabular floor which is an adverse, though not disqualifying, sign. We may reposition such hips up to about 14 years of age or later if specially indicated. Later still ankylosis or even arthrodesis in the correct functional position may be preferable if replacement is to be performed later.

(a) *Open reduction*

Hitherto the most serious problem has been the avoidance of reduction with undue tension, and attempts to overcome this by prolonged preliminary traction and soft-tissue release have not been notably successful, possibly because the hamstrings do not stretch and are seldom released. Femoral shortening at the time of open reduction together with extensive soft-tissue release renders these preliminary steps unnecessary (*Figure 2.14*).

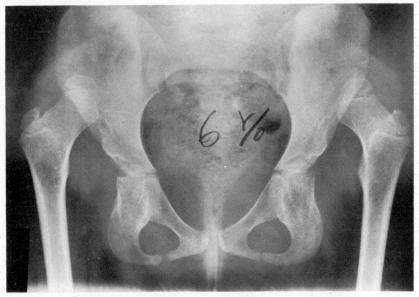

Figure 2.14. (a) High bilateral dislocations at the age of 8 years

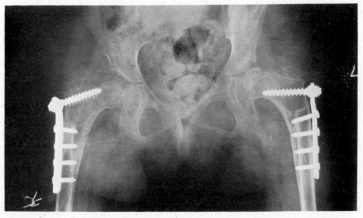

Figure 2.14. (b) Following open reduction and femoral shortening with varus and external rotation displacement

Open reduction with concurrent shortening has been largely developed in Central Europe by Gruca and Klisic (1975), Ashley, Larsen and James (1972) and is a most valuable adjuvant. Tension in the long pelvifemoral muscles and fascia is neutralized and, if the psoas tendon is divided and the glutei are released as far as possible posteriorly, compression on reduction may disappear, Furthermore, the proximal fragment is now fully mobile and may be widely abducted and distracted enabling the head to slip gently over the acetabular rim. Lastly, any difficulty in clearing obstructions from the acetabulum is overcome if its floor is approached through the osteotomy (*Figure 2.14*).

There are certain important technical considerations. The exposure must be wide, following the whole length of the iliac crest then turning downwards and backwards to the line of the femoral shaft along which it is extended. If the iliac apophysis is still cartilaginous it is split lengthwise and both the inner and outer surfaces of the ilium exposed subperiosteally from front to back. Sartorius and rectus femoris are detached anteriorly and the lateral surface of the femur is exposed by dissection between gluteus medius and tensor fascia. The fascia lata is cut transversely and split longitudinally together with the underlying vastus lateralis, the anterior half of which is displaced distally from its trochanteric origin. The psoas tendon is divided.

Acetabular clearance follows aided if necessary by exposure through a femoral osteotomy at the level of the lesser trochanter. The hip is reduced with the femoral fragments overlapping. The extent of this overlap controlled by gentle traction indicates the amount of femur to be removed which is usually about 1 inch. Redundant capsule is excised and reefed as in younger children and the wound closed with, on occasion, excision of part of the bony iliac crest to reduce tension on the suture line securing gluteus medius with the lateral half of the apophysis to the medial.

(b) *Stabilization of reduction*

Having made a femoral osteotomy it is natural that this should be used to correct any valgus or anteversion. Fixation is preferably performed by the Coventry method (*see* page 137) but a Rush nail may be used. If the latter is used there is a tendency for too much varus to occur during healing — a position acceptable in the young but less so in older children who have a shorter time to correct with growth. Furthermore, with nailing it will be necessary to secure the position of the hip joint. Two Kirschner wires are driven through the trochanter above the neck and on until visible within the pelvis. If placed through the head and acetabulum they may distract the joint. Similar fixation will sometimes be necessary when the Coventry method is used, for the extensive capsular dissection and excision may make adequate repair impossible.

The acetabulum may sometimes be remarkably well developed and the reduction stable, but in general it requires attention. The surgeon may choose between innominate re-alignment or acetabuloplasty using the excised femoral segment as a supporting graft. Having corrected anteversion, the head will be correctly placed beneath the reconstructed acetabular margin.

(c) *Salvage operations*

Failed open reduction in a young child indicates a second attempt with the knowledge that the result is likely to be less satisfactory than usual. The best time is within a few days of the original attempt but usually the true situation is not revealed until the plaster is removed. The causes of failure are numerous, ranging from failure to identify the true acetabulum to application of plaster carelessly or in the wrong position. Prompt diagnosis from a radiograph taken through plaster may be difficult when the head cannot be seen but the calcar is usually visible and its position in relation to the acetabulum identified. Sometimes when the head lies immediately in front of or behind the acetabulum it is even more difficult unless it is recognized that if a radiograph looks too good, i.e. the head is too deeply placed, it probably means that the hip remains dislocated. We must avoid procrastination, remove the plaster, repeat the radiograph and open the hip again for manipulation will certainly fail.

When redislocation is disclosed later the hip is usually stiff in abduction and it is best to wait until the hip is mobile again. The disaster of wound infection will prolong the waiting period in some indefinitely. There are three common patterns. First the hip remains totally dislocated, mobilization is rapid, the operation is simply an adequate open reduction and the outcome is more favourable. The cause may have been reduction into the false acetabulum, inadequate acetabular clearance, displacement during the application of plaster or failure to perform a necessary stabilizing operation. The femoral head usually remains spherical with its cartilage undamaged.

In contrast, we may find that the head has displaced from the acetabulum forwards or backwards. The situation is now quite different and far less favourable, for the head, having been compressed against the pelvis, is deformed, fixed by adhesions and covered with areas of cartilage loss which give a pockmarked appearance. Anterior dislocation is due to failure to appreciate acetabular anteversion and anterior deficiency which indicate careful capsular repair and stabilization by either innominate or femoral derotation osteotomy. Posterior dislocation is most commonly seen after innominate osteotomy which inevitably reduces stability posteriorly. Capsular plication and avoidance of excessive internal rotation will prevent this. Whether the dislocation is anterior or posterior the first essential is to mobilize the head by freeing adhesions and clearing the acetabulum of scar tissue. This may be tedious and difficult but femoral osteotomy provides not only a means of access from below, which greatly simplifies the problem, but allows correction of femoral deformity so providing one form of stabilization which may be used to reinforce a previous or concurrent acetabular operation. The most difficult are those in which an innominate osteotomy has been performed at the wrong level or with improper re-alignment.

Further indications for secondary open reduction arise when irreducible subluxation is allowed to develop with growth. A stabilizing operation will again be necessary, being directed towards the acetabulum, femur, or both, depending upon the anatomical state.

The Hey Groves—Colonna capsular arthroplasty (Colonna, 1953, 1965) has been superseded. Although the technique is demanding, this operation if correctly performed, is capable of giving satisfactory results in the 3—8-year age group but unfortunately beyond this the outcome is generally poor, for stiffness and deformity too frequently follow. The theoretical benefits are the ability to reduce tension by deepening the acetabulum upwards and medially which also overcomes any deficiency of acetabular development (*Figure 2.15*). Since the introduction of femoral shortening and improved methods of acetabular repair,

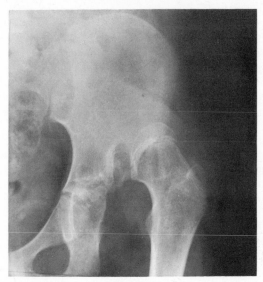

Figure 2.15. (a) Untreated unilateral dislocation at the age of 8 years

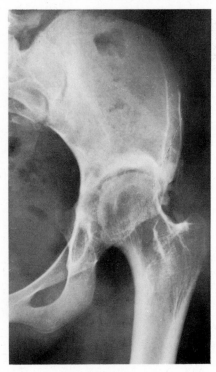

Figure 2.15. (b) 6 years later the hip remains in a partially reduced position and the joint space is maintained but the hip is stiff following Colonna arthroplasty

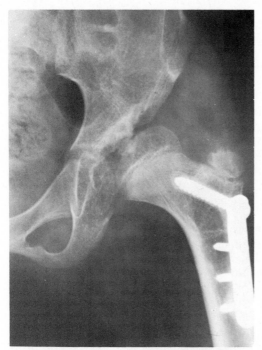
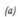

Figure 2.16. (a) At 7 years the acetabulum has failed to develop and there is subluxation. (b) Chiari's osteotomy performed. (c) The appearance 4 years later

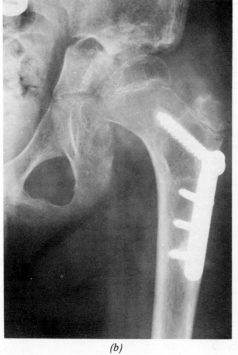

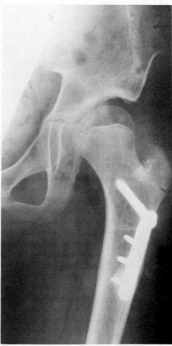

there is little temptation to employ this damaging operation even within the recommended age range, let alone in older children for whom, if not so unpredictable, this might well have been a useful alternative in some patients. Irreducible subluxation is another possible indication but Chiari's pelvic osteotomy is to be preferred.

Pelvic osteotomy (Chiari, 1955) is well described by Colton (1972) in English. This method is an important contribution to the treatment of primary or secondary subluxation at an age when reduction is neither possible nor desirable because of deformity of the head or acetabulum with or without secondary degenerative changes and pain. There are, of course, limitations governed by the degree of upward displacement for, clearly, the osteotomy must not enter the sacro-iliac joint. As in Salter's innominate osteotomy, attention to details of technique is essential to success.

This operation supersedes the high-shelf for two reasons. Firstly, union of the transverse supra-acetabular pelvic osteotomy is rapid and there is no unsupported graft to break or absorb. Secondly, medial displacement of the femoral head and acetabulum reduces the load on the hip joint imposed by the abductor lever. This is further reduced when a varus derotation femoral osteotomy is performed concurrently. This is frequently necessary if the head is to lie beneath the centre of the superior pelvic buttress.

Common errors in technique include an osteotomy which inclines downwards thus preventing medial displacement. Displacement may be too little when support is inadequate or too much when there is instability and limited bone contact which delays union. The distal fragment may even slip backwards. The osteotomy itself may be too high or too low. The former is preferable for if not excessive the gap will subsequently fill with bone whereas, if too low, compression and stiffness may follow. Chiari's 'closed' approach with radiographic control may not appeal to the surgeon inexperienced in the operation, so that wide exposure enabling the osteotomy to be performed under direct vision is probably preferable.

When contemplating Chiari's osteotomy for the first time it is prudent to perform it on a cadaver beforehand — a recommendation which applies equally to Salter's operation. When correctly indicated and performed, satisfactory results in about 75 per cent of patients are being increasingly reported from many centres. This is encouraging for the hip joint to which it is applicable is likely otherwise to fail in early adult life (*Figure 2.16*).

Arthrodesis This is today in disrepute, especially for girls, but it may be the ultimate salvage operation for otherwise irreparable and painful unilateral dislocations. The functional and cosmetic result may be excellent in men and it should be possible to perform replacement arthroplasty if necessary later. The Pyrford technique (Apley and Denham, 1955) is admirable for femoral osteotomy permits arthrodesis at the correct level in the position which gives the best contact. The position of the leg is then adjusted at the osteotomy with some overlap which if excessive may be corrected by resection. The youth of these patients ensures a high incidence of fusion.

Abduction osteotomy and gluteal advancement   These combined or as alterna-tives, will alleviate the problem when the capital growth plate has closed prematurely. The result is a short varus neck and proximal overgrowth of the greater trochanter causing a block to abduction and gluteal insufficiency (*see* page 50). Such hips are usually congruous and, providing this is confirmed in adduction, an abduction osteotomy is indicated. If the acetabulum is deficient but stable, distal displacement of the trochanter with its gluteal attachment will be preferred. We may add some form of acetabular stabilizing operation if there is any instability.

MISCELLANEOUS OBSERVATIONS ON THE CLINICAL AND RADIOLOGICAL FEATURES

Much of the foregoing description of assessment and indications has been concerned with radiographic appearances but we must not neglect the significance of physical signs at all stages of management.

We have already considered in some detail the diagnostic significance of the signs found on examination of the newborn. As the child develops, diagnosis of unilateral dislocation will depend upon the recognition of a loss of abduction in flexion and unilateral shortening when, with hips and knees flexed and feet together, the knee levels are compared. When walking begins, and this is seldom unduly delayed, the gait is characteristic and quite specific. The foot on the dislocated side is placed flat on the ground and the opposite knee is flexed to compensate for shortening (*Figure 2.17*). If shortening is due to other causes and the hip is stable, compensation is achieved by equinus on the shorter side. The Trendelenburg gait may not appear until the child is two years old.

When dislocation is bilateral, these signs are not present and the difficulties of diagnosis are consequently greater. There is great variability between normal children in the range of abduction in flexion but if this is less than 45° we may suspect symmetrical abnormality which may be dislocation or possibly infantile coxa vara, Perthes' disease, spastic diplegia or some generalized disorder such as dysplasia multiplex epiphysialis. Palpation of elevated greater trochanters and widening of the pelvis will augment suspicion but a radiograph is now essential. When walking begins, we have no specific diagnostic sign to help us for the lumbar lordosis characteristic of bilateral dislocation is equally a feature of the toddler's gait. The Trendelenburg gait is again delayed.

Although joint laxity may be an important factor in aetiology it is also significant as an influence obscuring diagnosis. Laxity may neutralize the mech-anical block to abduction so that this important sign is less readily elicited. In unilateral dislocation this is still likely to be detectable in the placid child as a slight difference in both the range and rhythm of abduction and the contours of the thigh, but this is only detected with difficulty in the recalcitrant (*Figure 2.18*). When the dislocation is bilateral the diagnosis may be exceedingly difficult. Hypotonia and other neuromuscular disorders have a similar influence on diagnosis with the added disadvantage that the stability of primary reduction may be compromised.

Palpating the head of the femur has an important role under two circum-stances. First, we may confirm that apparently successful primary reduction by

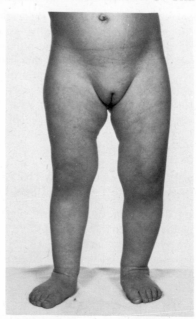

Figure 2.17. The right hip is dislocated and the child stands with the left knee flexed

traction as seen on the radiograph has in fact been achieved. It is easy to confuse this with anterior reposition so that clinical examination should not be neglected at this stage. Later, a radiograph may be judged to be satisfactory when in fact the femoral head is lying immediately in front of or behind the acetabulum. Palpation will resolve the problem by detecting undue prominence of the head or its absence from its normal position. Suspicion will be reinforced by discovering restricted medial rotation in anterior displacement and lateral rotation in the posterior.

Although dislocation of the hip may be a component of several syndromes, such as Larsen's, Freeman–Sheldon, Ehlers–Danlos and others including arthrogryposis, we must be particularly alert to the possibilities of underlying neuromuscular disease. The association of hip dislocation with other deformities of the leg, notably talipes equinovarus (calcaneovalgus is an exception), is a warning sign. Failure to maintain a successful primary reduction is another. We must now remember the congenital myopathies of varying severity and prognosis, cerebral palsy and myelodysplasia or spinal dysraphism.

There will be few problems in radiological interpretation if a simple philosophy is adopted. The radiograph either reveals an entirely satisfactory situation, i.e. congruous concentric reduction (in abduction at first and later in the neutral position), or it must be interpreted as entirely unsatisfactory. If unsatisfactory, there is usually a lateral or upward displacement of the head but occasionally the head may appear too deeply contained. This implies that it lies immediately in front of or behind the acetabulum. Special views or techniques are seldom absolutely necessary except when it is desirable to establish whether congruity

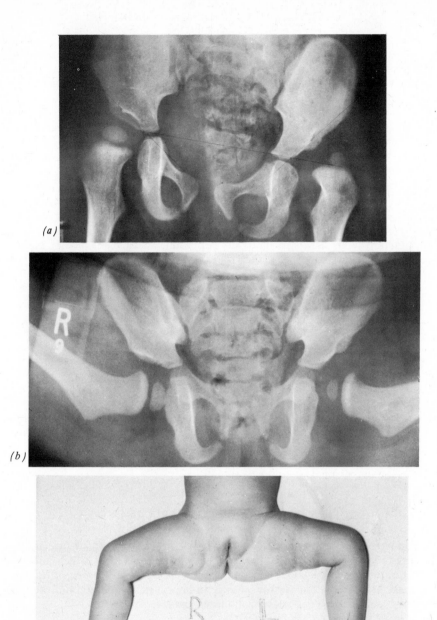

(a)

(b)

(c)

Figure 2.18. (a) Dislocation on the left and considerable subluxation on the right.
(b) In full abduction congruity is restored on the right but there is some persistent
lying away on the left. (c) To illustrate the degree of abduction obtained to produce
the x-ray illustrated in (b)

of the hip can be restored by positioning of the leg (*see* page 81). Lateral projections will confirm anterior or posterior reposition but stress or standing radiographs and abduction views in neonatal diagnosis add little to the information obtainable from routine methods coupled with clinical examination.

It is always essential to appreciate that the hip joint is almost entirely cartilaginous, and therefore translucent, in young children. Estimations of acetabular angles are therefore of little value before the age of four or five years, and of none whatsoever if the pelvis is askew in the sagittal or coronal plane.

An arthrogram will outline the cartilaginous structures but provides little information of prognostic value for subsequent acetabular development is dependent more upon the maintenance of concentric reduction than the profile of the cartilaginous acetabulum at any one time. This aspect was investigated at The Hospital for Sick Children by Sallis and Smith (1965) (Table 2.II) (*see* page 68).

Arthrography has its partisans and is certainly valuable as a method of documentation and a tool of clinical research (Somerville and Scott, 1957). If, however, the proposition expressed at the beginning of this section is followed faithfully and the hip is explored when congruity is imperfect, arthrography does no more than anticipate certain likely operative findings. There is, nevertheless, one situation in which this investigation is valuable. When we have apparently reduced the hip by traction in a child of around one year of age, the quality of reduction may be difficult to assess because of the translucency of the vital structures. When some lateral displacement is present we are uncertain whether this is due to anteversion, which will probably resolve, or an obstruction, which at this age is likely to be the acetabular labrum (limbus).

Although obstruction due to this will usually disappear if submitted to the continuing pressure of the femoral head in abduction (Severin, 1950) (*Figure 2.8*), this method of resolving the problem is less desirable than surgical removal. This is because some degree of compression will be imposed upon both the femoral head, which may cause deformity, and also upon the periphery of the acetabulum, thereby inhibiting its growth.

PRIMARY SUBLUXATION (ACETABULAR DYSPLASIA)

Although this may be regarded as no more than a forme fruste of congenital dislocation there are certain features specific to this variety which justify its separate consideration. A clear distinction must be made between primary and secondary subluxation for the latter is an important complication of the treatment of dislocation and has been discussed already.

Clinical features

The detection of primary subluxation during the first year often occurs by chance when a radiograph is taken for some other reason. At this stage there are no abnormal physical signs to help us unless abduction in flexion is limited at extreme range. The hip is unlikely to be unstable and the clunk sign may be absent or not detectable after the first few days of life. However, it should be

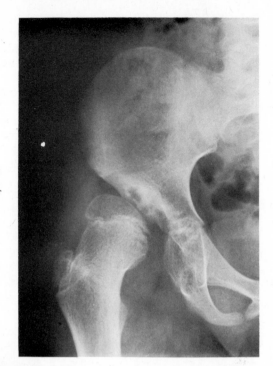

Figure 2.19. (a) There is a severe upward subluxation and acetabular insufficiency at the age of 9 years

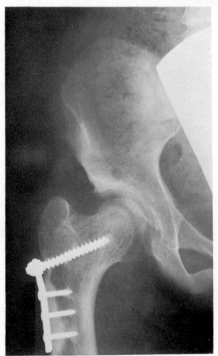

Figure 2.19. (b) 5 years after open reduction, acetabuloplasty and femoral osteotomy

with the object of detecting acetabular dysplasia that a radiograph should be taken of spontaneously stabilizing hips at 4 and 12 months of age. As previously emphasized, we must beware of interpreting as acetabular dysplasia the apparent inadequacy of pelvic obliquity which is an artefact. We will, however, remain alert to the possibility of true dysplasia arising secondary to persisting pelvic obliquity more particularly if it is associated with infantile idiopathic scoliosis which may be either progressive or slower than usual to resolve.

When walking begins, limitation of abduction becomes more readily identifiable if looked for in a child with a slightly asymmetrical gait. Still later, a limp develops and we may frequently be told that this appeared at a certain time on a certain day which suggests that earlier stability has suddenly given way. Later still, the older child may present with a limp and some pain as the first indication that all is not well. Although bilateral primary subluxation is unusual, contra-lateral subluxation is commonly seen in association with dislocation when diagnosis and management are dominated by the more affected side.

Lastly, the prognosis for undetected or uncorrected subluxation is poor for osteoarthritis develops early and is often disabling — more so in fact and earlier than in untreated dislocation. It is possible that 20 per cent of osteoarthritic hips are attributable to this malformation (Lloyd-Roberts, 1955). We must therefore increase our efforts to diagnose early and treat vigorously.

Anatomy

Upward subluxation has a more serious effect on acetabular development than complete dislocation for the cartilaginous lip of the acetabulum is, to a degree which varies with displacement, subjected to pressure and its growth is thereby inhibited (*Figure 2.19*). This is in contrast to dislocation in which, although deprived of the stimulus of weight-bearing, the acetabulum is not so compressed and thus its capacity to develop when given the appropriate stimulus is greater and persists longer. This is the fundamental anatomical feature of subluxation. The compression between head and acetabulum also has an effect upon the capital epiphysis which will be indented or flattened at the point of contact.

The other changes are secondary and of less significance in the early stages. Upward movement inevitably increases the distance between the inferior segment of the head and the non-articular floor of the acetabulum. This is occupied by soft tissue, i.e. the fat pad and a fold of capsule drawn up into the cavity. At this stage it is still possible to restore congruity by positioning the hip in abduction and internal rotation, but later this becomes impossible, for the capsular fold adheres to the acetabular floor and to the transverse ligament beneath which the ligamentum teres passes. Furthermore, the ligamentum teres itself lengthens and thickens to cause an additional obstruction. Later still, the ilio-psoas shortens.

Femoral-neck anteversion with some valgus are likely accompaniments and they reinforce the tendency to subluxation. However, femoral and acetabular anteversion will tend to maintain a closer relationship than in dislocation. The joint will, nonetheless, tend to lie abnormally far forward and the anterior segment of the head will be relatively uncovered so that it is more readily palpable beneath the inguinal ligament.

PRIMARY SUBLUXATION (ACETABULAR DYSPLASIA)

Radiological features in relation to treatment

Although it is customary to calculate the acetabular angle by Hilgenriener's method (*see* page 68) and express an opinion upon the degree of acetabular maldevelopment, this is seldom contributory in early childhood. There are several reasons for this. Firstly, the true acetabular lip, being cartilaginous, is translucent, and secondly, it is often difficult to obtain a well centred radiograph at this age — and any variation in lateral tilt or rotation at the pelvis will greatly modify the reading. Lastly, standards of normality are less reliable in the very young in contrast to the older child when we say that an angle in excess of 20° is abnormal.

It is far more important to study the relationship between the head and acetabulum and the integrity of Shenton's line. Before walking begins, the femoral head will frequently appear to lie too far laterally in relation to the acetabular floor and this is accentuated if there is delay in walking due to hypotonia and joint laxity. Providing that Shenton's line remains intact or, if minimally breached, is restored by abducting the hip, and providing there is no delay in epiphyseal ossification and no limitation of abduction on clinical examination, then no action is necessary except surveillance by serial radiographs. This appearance is not due to hip joint dysplasia as such but rather persistence of fetal alignment (anteversion) of the femur which is usually rapidly adjusted when weight is taken and the glutei develop functional activity. The corollary is that a significant breach in Shenton's line, coupled with some lateral displacement of the femoral epiphysis with delay in ossification, and limitation of abduction even at extreme range on one side, constitute the signs upon which we base the diagnosis in the young child of between 4 and 12 months of age.

At less than 4 months, when the capital epiphysis is normally translucent, clinical signs or a history of instability at birth are more significant in diagnosis than radiological evidence. As growth proceeds, the radiological diagnosis becomes obvious, until finally the signs so characteristic of neglected subluxation in the mature hip are evident. These include, in addition to displacement, a deformed head, acetabular deficiency with an exostosis in the non-articular area, and thickening of the bone on the inferior border of the neck (Wiberg, 1939).

Management of primary subluxation

The method employed depends upon the possibility of restoring congruity of the hip by positioning the leg in abduction and internal rotation.

(a) If congruity is restored, action depends upon the age of the child — if walking has not begun it is unlikely that significant upward displacement, and therefore acetabular lip compression, will have occurred. It would seem proper, therefore, to start by using an abduction splint to maintain congruity within the acetabulum, providing that the stimulating effect of movement without compression is maintained and there is no tension in the adductor muscles when the splint is applied. The Denis Browne hip harness (which has been described) is ideal for it allows controlled movement of the hip and mobility of the child. It is essential, however, that no force is used when abducting the hips to apply the harness. Such force exposes the epiphysis to the risk of ischaemia and should be avoided by a preliminary adductor tenotomy. Within 4 to 6 months most subluxations will be corrected and the acetabulum will show evidence of satisfactory development.

When the harness is removed it is important to confirm that congruity is maintained in the erect weight-bearing position. If not, congruity will need to be stabilized by either an innominate or femoral varus and external rotation osteotomy as in the dislocated hip.

Children who are walking are better treated by immediate osteotomy of one or other variety. They will probably have rather more displacement and their acetabulae may well have suffered some compression. The sooner compression is relieved and the normal stimulus of weight-bearing erect is restored the better. Furthermore, they are intolerant of the restraint of a splint, once having experienced the pleasures of independence.

In any event, supervision must continue until maturity is reached lest there is a recurrence of subluxation or a later failure of acetabular growth. Some of these aspects and the relative value and technique of the two types of osteotomy have already been considered in relation to treatment of dislocation.

(b) When congruity cannot be restored by positioning, the management is that of congenital dislocation, for without congruity neither innominate nor femoral osteotomy alone can be effective. These patients occupy the border-line between subluxation and dislocation and in both restoration of congruity is the first essential by means of traction, open reduction, or both. We must resist the temptation to compromise and be constantly aware of the distinction between reducible and irreducible subluxations.

Even when traction succeeds in reducing the subluxation we must remember that the acetabulum has been compressed and that some form of reconstruction or re-alignment will be needed, not necessarily immediately, but in the future, if acetabular growth fails. If subluxation persists and open reduction is necessary, special attention must be directed to the floor of the acetabulum where the obstruction to reduction is usually found. We will be prepared to deepen the acetabulum at an earlier age and with less structural dysplasia than in patients with dislocation. Furthermore, reduction demands far less anatomical rearrangement with, in consequence, less risk to the epiphyseal blood supply. We may therefore proceed to concurrent femoral osteotomy without undue anxiety, if excessive anteversion is present. This is most likely to be necessary when acetabuloplasty is preferred to acetabular re-alignment in order to place the epiphysis beneath the deepened segment of the rim (*Figure 2.19*).

(c) Older children with irreducible subluxation, epiphyseal deformity and secondary changes in the floor of the acetabulum are difficult to manage. Although it may be technically possible to reduce the hip, this may be of little benefit if there are secondary deformities of the articulating surfaces. A further difficulty arises when, as is often the case, there is no pain and movements are free, for there is a danger of producing functional deterior-

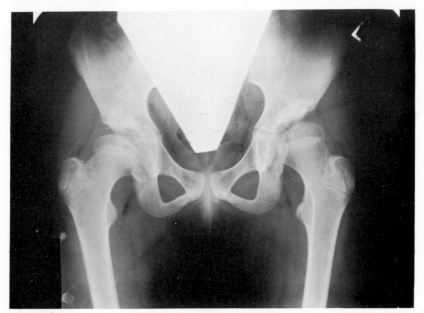

Figure 2.20. (a) There is severe acetabular insufficiency with only slight upward subluxation

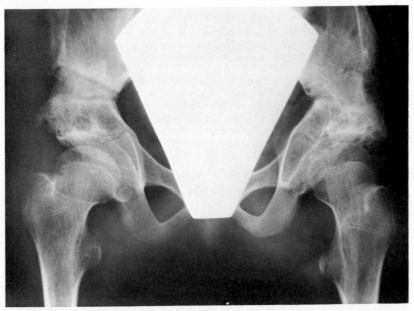

Figure 2.20. (b) Soon after innominate osteotomy to show considerable improvement in acetabular contour

ation without significantly reducing the prospect of degenerative changes later. In most it is better to accept the situation so long as there is no pain. When pain obtrudes, Chiari's pelvic osteotomy, often accompanied by femoral derotation, is clearly indicated (*Figure 2.16*).

(d) Acetabular dysplasia without subluxation is the least common presentation. This may be discovered by chance in the older child or unexpectedly follow earlier successful correction of subluxation of a degree, and at an age, when acetabular reconstruction was judged to be unnecessary. In these circumstances Salter's innominate osteotomy is clearly indicated and consistently successful (*Figure 2.20*).

Subluxation should not be regarded merely as a minor variety of dislocation and treated with correspondingly reduced vigour. There are problems peculiar to it which in some respects make management more difficult and our results may be less satisfactory than those that we expect to achieve in dislocated hips. Furthermore, the penalty of failure is often disabling osteoarthritis in early adult life which contrasts with the long pain-free interval which characterizes untreated dislocation. Lastly, if dislocation is converted to subluxation by inadequate treatment, the prognosis is even worse than that of primary subluxation.

REFERENCES

Andren, L. and Borglin, N. E. (1961). Disturbed urinary excretion pattern of oestrogens in newborns with congenital dislocation of the hip. 1. The excretion of oestrogen during the first few days of life. *Acta endocr. Copenh.* **37**, 423

Apley, A. G. and Denham, R. A. (1955). Osteotomy as an aid to arthrodesis of the hip. *J. Bone Jt Surg.* **37B**, 185

Ashley, R. K., Larsen, L. U. and James, P. M. (1972). Reduction of dislocation of the hip in older children. A preliminary report. *J. Bone Jt Surg.* **54A**, 545

Badgley, C. E. and O'Connor, S. J. (1953). The clinical significance of retention of foetal position of the limb. Proceedings of the American Acadamy of Orthopaedic Surgeons. *J. Bone Jt Surg.* **35A**, 498

Barlow, T. G. (1962). Early diagnosis and treatment of congenital dislocation of the hip. *J. Bone Jt Surg.* **44B**, 292

Barlow, T. G. (1966). Congenital dislocation of the hip in the newborn. Early diagnosis and treatment of congenital dislocation of the hip in the newborn. *Proc. R. Soc. Med.* **59**, 1103

Borring, T. D. J., and Scrase, W. H. (1965). Premature epiphyseal fusion at the knee complicating prolonged immobilisation for congenital dislocation of the hip. *J. Bone Jt Surg.* **47B**, 280

Browne, D. (1936). Congenital deformities of mechanical origin. *Proc. R. Soc. Med.* (Section for the study of Disease in Children). **29**, 1409

Carter, C. O. and Wilkinson, J. A. (1964). Persistent joint laxity and congenital dislocation of the hip. *J. Bone Jt Surg.* **46B**, 40

Catterall, A. (1977). In preparation

Chiari, K. (1955). Ergelonisse mit der Beckenosteotomie als Pfannendachplastik. *Z. Orthop.* **87**, 14

Colonna, P. C. (1953). Capsular arthroplasty for congenital dislocation of the hip. A two-stage procedure. *J. Bone Jt Surg.* **35A**, 179

Colonna, P. C. (1965). Capsular arthroplasty for congenital dislocation of the hip. Indications and technique. Some long-term results. *J. Bone Jt Surg.* **47A**, 437

Colton, C. L. (1972). Chiari osteotomy for acetabular dysplasia in young subjects. *J. Bone Jt Surg.* **54B**, 579

Cook, E. J., and Pilcher, M. F. (1977). In preparation

REFERENCES

Dunn, P. M. (1969). Congenital dislocation of the hip (C.D.H.). Necropsy studies at birth. *Proc. R. Soc. Med.* **62**, 1035

Finlay, H. U. L., Maudsley, R. H. and Busfield, P. I. (1967). Dislocated hip in the newborn infant. *Br. Med. J.* **IV**, 377

Harris, N., Catterall, A., and Lloyd-Roberts, G. C. (1976). In preparation

Harris, N. H., Lloyd-Roberts, and Gallien, R. (1975). Acetabular development in congenital dislocation of the hip. *J. Bone Jt Surg.* **57B**, 46

Klisic, Y. (1975). Personal communication

Le Damany, P. (1908). Die angeboure Hüftgelenksverrenkung. *Z. Orthop. Chir.* **21**, 129

Lloyd-Roberts, G. C. (1955). Osteoarthritis of the hip: a study of clinical pathology. *J. Bone Jt Surg.* **37B**, 8

Lloyd-Roberts, G. C. and Pilcher, M. F. (1965). Structural idiopathic scoliosis in infancy: a study of the natural history of 100 patients. *J. Bone Jt Surg.* **47B**, 520

Lloyd-Roberts, G. C. and Swann, M. (1966). Pitfalls in the management of congenital dislocation of the hip. *J. Bone Jt Surg.* **48B**, 666

MacKenzie, I. G. (1972). Congenital dislocation of the hip. The development of a regional service. *J. Bone Jt Surg.* **54B**, 18

MacKenzie, I. G., Seddon, H. J. and Trevor, D. (1960). Congenital dislocation of the hip. *J. Bone Jt Surg.* **42B**, 689

McKibbin, B. (1970). Anatomical factors in the stability of the hip joint in the newborn. *J. Bone Jt Surg.* **52B**, 148

Mau, H., Dörr, W. M., Henkel, L., and Lutsche, J. (1971). Open reduction of congenital dislocation of the hip by Ludloff's method. *J. Bone Jt Surg.* **53A**, 1281

Mitchell, G. P. (1972). Problems in the early diagnosis and management of congenital dislocation of the hip. *J. Bone Jt Surg.* **54B**, 4

Nelson, M. A. (1966). Early diagnosis of congenital dislocation of the hip. *J. Bone Jt Surg.* **48B**, 388

Ortolani, M. (1937). Un segno poco noto e sua importanza per la diagnosi precoce di prelussazione congenita dell'anca. *La Pediatria* **45**, 129

Palmen, K. (1961). Preluxation of the hip joint. *Acta Paediatrica* **50**, suppl. 129

Ralis, Z. and McKibbin, B. (1973). Changes in shape of the human hip joint during its development and their relation to its stability. *J. Bone Jt Surg.* **55B**, 780

Rosen, S. Von (1962). Diagnosis and treatment of congenital dislocation of the hip joint in the newborn. *J. Bone Jt Surg.* **44B**, 284

Rosen, S. Von (1968). Further experience with congenital dislocation of the hip in the newborn. *J. Bone Jt Surg.* **50B**, 538

Sallis, J. G. and Smith, R. G. (1965). A study of the development of the acetabular roof in congenital dislocation of the hip. *Br. J. Surg.* **52**, 44

Salter, R. B. (1966). Role of innominate osteotomy in the treatment of congenital dislocation and subluxation of the hip in the older child. *J. Bone Jt Surg.* **48A**, 1413

Salter, R. B. (1967). C.D.H. In *Modern Trends in Orthopaedics*, No. 5. Ed. W. D. Graham New York: Appleton-Century-Crofts

Scaglietti, O. and Calandriello, B. (1962). Open reduction of congenital dislocation of the hip. *J. Bone Jt Surg.* **44B**, 257

Scott, J. C. (1953). Frame reduction in C.D.H. *J. Bone Jt Surg.* **35B**, 372

Severin, E. (1941). Contribution to the knowledge of congenital dislocation of the hip joints; late results of closed reduction and arthrographic studies of recent cases. *Acta Chir. Scand.* **84, suppl. 63**, 1

Severin, E. (1950). Congenital dislocation of the hip. Development of the joint after closed reduction. *J. Bone Jt Surg.* **32A**, 507

Small, G. B. (1968). Congenital dislocation of the hip in the newborn. *J. Bone Jt Surg.* **50B**, 524

Somerville, E. W. (1953). Development of congenital dislocation of the hip. *J. Bone Jt Surg.* **35B**, 568

Somerville, E. W. (1967). Results of treatment of 100 congenitally dislocated hips. *J. Bone Jt Surg.* **49B**, 258

Somerville, E. W. (1974). The nature of the congenitally dislocated hip. *Proc. R. Soc. Med.* **67**, 1169

REFERENCES

Somerville, E. W. and Scott, J. C. (1957). The direct approach to congenital dislocation of the hip. *J. Bone Jt Surg.* **39B,** 623

Stanisavljevic S. and Mitchell, C. L. (1963). Congenital dysplasia, subluxation and dislocation of the hip in stillborn and newborn infants. *J. Bone Jt Surg.* **45A,** 1147

Steele, H. (1973). Triple osteotomy of the innominate bone. *J. Bone Jt Surg.* **55A,** 343

Trevor, D. (1957). Treatment of C.D.H. *J. Bone Jt Surg.* **39B,** 611

Trevor, D., Johns, D. L. and Fixsen, J. A. (1975). Acetabuloplasty in the treatment of C.D.H. *J. Bone Jt Surg.* **57B,** 167

Trueta, J. (1957). The normal vascular anatomy of the human femoral head during growth. *J. Bone Jt Surg.* **39B,** 358

Weissman, S. L. (1954). Congenital dysplasia of the hip. Observations on the 'normal' joint in cases of unilateral disease. *J. Bone Jt Surg.* **36B,** 385

Wiberg, G. (1939). Studies on dysplastic acetabula and congenital subluxation of the hip joint. *Acta Chir. Scand.* **Suppl. 58**

Wilkinson, J. A. (1963). Prime factors in the aetiology of congenital dislocation of the hip. *J. Bone Jt Surg.* **45B,** 268

Wilkinson, J. A. (1972). A post-natal survey for congenital displacement of the hip. *J. Bone Jt Surg.* **54B,** 40

Wilkinson, J. and Carter, C. (1960). Congenital dislocation of the hip. The results of conservative treatment. *J. Bone Jt Surg.* **42B,** 669

Williamson, Jean (1972). Difficulties of early diagnosis and treatment of congenital dislocation of the hip in Northern Ireland. *J. Bone Jt Surg.* **54B,** 13

Wynne-Davies, Ruth (1970). Acetabular dysplasia and familial joint laxity. Two aetiological factors in congenital dislocation of the hip. A review of 589 patients and their families. *J. Bone Jt Surg.* **52B,** 704

3

Pyogenic Arthritis of the Hip

G. C. Lloyd-Roberts

There are two distinct varieties distinguished by and related to the age of onset. Disease arising within the neonatal period of the first year differs in almost every respect from that in the older child, whose age at infection coincides with that of the highest incidence of osteomyelitis namely, 5 to 10 years. They will be considered separately.

PYOGENIC ARTHRITIS OF INFANCY

Rapid destruction is the most striking feature (*Figure 3.1*). This reflects the great vulnerability of cartilage, of which the joint is largely composed, to pyogenic organisms. The manner of destruction is not, however, just a simple matter of bacterial invasion delivering a direct attack, nor of digestion through the agency of infected synovial pannus, (which is a relatively slow process), but involves more subtle mechanisms, involving the anatomy of the blood supply, the properties of pyogenic pus and the immunological efficiency of the patient.

(a) The blood supply to the capital epiphysis in infancy differs from that in the older child in that the vessels from the metaphyseal area penetrate the growth plate to enter the epiphysis. They have no barrier until ossification begins on the epiphyseal side of the plate. This provides a ready-made channel for both the spread of infection to the epiphysis and a pre-disposition to ischaemic necrosis if thrombosis occurs. This combination alone may be lethal to the epiphysis and the growth plate (Trueta, 1959).

(b) Pyogenic pus has certain properties which are injurious to cartilage. This was observed by Phemister (1924) and ascribed to the action of proteolytic ferments derived from degenerating polymorphonuclear cells. Lack (1959) has investigated this proposition and proposes that plasminogen normally present in the blood is activated by a kinase derived from pyogenic bacteria to produce plasmin. The normal role of plasmin is to remove excess fibrin but if it is itself in excess it will digest the mucoprotein of cartilage overcoming the action of its own inhibitor.

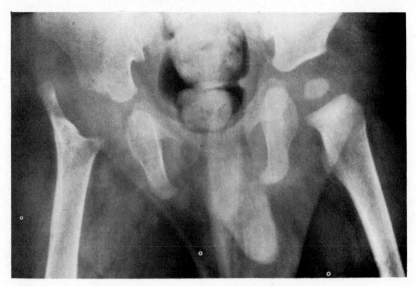

Figure 3.1. The head and neck of the femur are apparently destroyed

(c) Immunodeficiency is characterized by a subdued clinical response to infection which is a feature of neonatal pyogenic arthritis and may account for delay in diagnosis. We have recently investigated this association (Kuo *et al.*, 1975) and have found that more than half of all our patients had evidence of abnormality of immunoglobulins, complement or phagocytes. We would expect a relative hypofunction of immune mechanisms in the neonate, especially in the premature, and indeed three patients studied at the time of the initial infection confirmed this suspicion. However the persistence of some degree of immunodeficiency in 6 of 12 studied retrospectively suggests that the defective mechanism is of greater significance than a transitory physiological phenomenon. Indeed, low IgA recordings were found in patients up to the age of 16 years (Table 3.1).

TABLE 3.I

Six children with septic arthritis in infancy and low plasma IgA levels on review

Age at onset (days)	Premature	Culture	Age at review (years)
27	–	Staphylococcus	16
35	–	Staphylococcus	15
21	Yes	Staphylococcus	9
180	–	Staphylococcus	3
11	Yes	Staphylococcus	1½
14	Yes	Staphylococcus	1½

The practical implication, apart from a deceptively mild clinical response, is some failure of resistance to the spread of infection and consequently a greater extent of destruction. Thus 5 of 6 patients with total loss of the femoral head had low levels of IgA whereas 3 of 4 with partial loss had normal levels. Furthermore, the incidence of wound infection following reconstructive operations was also related to these levels so that adequate antibiotic cover, full blood substitution and careful dissection and haemostasis become even more important than usual.

Bacteriology

Staphylococcus aureus is now the predominant invader, whereas in the past streptococci were found almost as frequently. Antibiotic sensitivity would seem to explain this. A wide range of bacteria has however been described. The portal of entry is usually from a focus of metaphyseal osteomyelitis secondary to septicaemia arising from a failure to contain infection of the skin, throat or elsewhere. There are, however, two alternative pathways peculiar to the newborn: firstly, via the umbilicus with its inevitable vulnerability to infection and drained by remnants of the fetal circulation, and secondly, as a result of femoral venepuncture so commonly employed at this age (Chacha, 1971). The needle, which may so readily pass through the vein and enter the hip, may either infect directly or, by causing a haemarthrosis, provide a localizing medium for any circulating bacteria.

Clinical diagnosis

The baby may be either very ill or unexpectedly unaffected by the severe illness. Both presentations tend to obscure the diagnosis. If the baby is prostrate, flaccid, rejecting or vomiting feeds, icteric, cyanosed or convulsing, attention will be concentrated on the whole rather than the part. If, on the other hand, the manifestation is one of mild unexplained fever, feeding difficulty and failure to thrive, it is difficult to believe that this is the constitutional response to a severe destructive infection. Awareness and suspicion are the basis upon which the correct diagnosis is made (Obletz, 1960).

Local examination may also fail to reveal the true nature of the problem in the early stages, especially if antibiotics have masked the signs. There may be little more than a disinclination to move or a pain reaction on passive movement. The hip will, however, rapidly adopt a flexed and adducted posture, and oedema, affecting particularly the adductor region and genitalia, will appear. Signs of an abscess and hip displacement may develop later and imply that destruction has probably proceded beyond the stage of potential recovery.

In neonatal life there is, for practical purposes, no differential diagnosis of the local lesion. Birth fractures in this region are rare except in osteogenesis imperfecta. Congenital syphilis is now of historical interest only and some conditions such as scurvy are prevented by the transmission of deficiency factors through the maternal circulation. Later, however, we must consider assault, Caffey's cortical hyperostosis (rare in this situation) and neurological or idiopathic dislocation in addition to metabolic, deficiency, haematological and neoplastic disease.

Radiological features

The first sign is swelling due to oedema within the soft tissues. Much play is made of capsular distension but Brown (1975) has shown from this hospital that the so-called capsular line is an intermuscular plane which varies in position with that of the leg. This line however will be more prominent when there is oedema within the surrounding muscles.

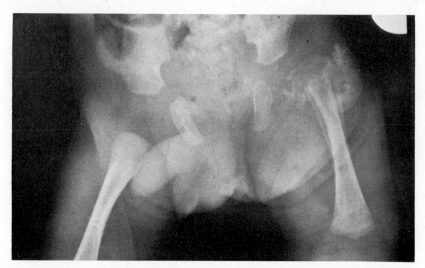

Figure 3.2. The vigorous periosteal reaction is characteristic in the early stages

Periostitis around the proximal femoral shaft may appear within three days of the onset in contrast to the delay in older children. Its early appearance and situation suggest that the primary focus is within the bone rather than the joint. Periostitis may rapidly become exuberant (*Figure 3.2*).

The head and neck are unossified and translucent so we will not see changes in this area unless the hip dislocates or there is displacement at the level of a pathological fracture of the neck. These are, of course, signs of tardy diagnosis and indicate that the hip is so damaged that we cannot expect to achieve a good final result.

During the months that follow, ossification is delayed and translucency persists. At 1 year we are in a quandary if there is no displacement for we do not know whether the proximal femur is truly in continuity with the hip, or whether a hitherto stable pseudarthrosis intervenes. Displacement will, of course, mean either dislocation of the hip without pseudarthrosis, an unstable pseudarthrosis or destruction of the femoral component of the hip. This appearance is too often interpreted as indicating destruction alone and no action is taken. Ossification within the remaining cartilage will ultimately disclose the true nature of the deformity when the most favourable time to intervene will have passed (Lloyd-Roberts, 1960). It is tempting to employ arthrography to resolve the dilemma but intra-articular adhesions confuse interpretation and little additional information is obtained. Arthrography is no substitute for exploration, the technique and findings of which will be discussed when treatment is considered, together with a further description of the morbid anatomy.

Lastly, we must enlarge upon the mechanism of persisting translucency when there is, in fact, continuity of cartilage. This is best studied at the knee which is

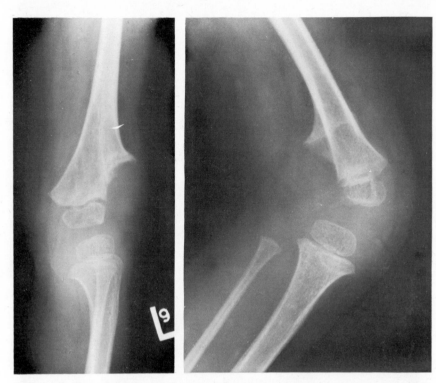

Figure 3.3. The epiphysis, growth plate and metaphysis appear to have been partially destroyed in both the anterior and lateral projections

easily examined. The radiograph may suggest that half the epiphysis, its underlying growth plate and the nearby metaphysis are destroyed (*Figure 3.3*) Clinically, however, the knee is mobile, relatively stable and the 'missing' condyle is palpable (*Figure 3.4*). Ossification will slowly advance to invade this area and the final outcome may be surprisingly good (*Figure 3.5*). No harm is done by failing to recognize this situation early on for the knee is, and remains, stable without displacement and no surgical treatment is indicated. The hip differs in that we cannot examine it as efficiently and inactivity may greatly prejudice the outcome.

Persisting translucency, if not indicating destruction, is probably due to one of three factors: firstly, the osteoporosis of the acute infection; secondly, damage to the germinal cells of the growth plate and capital epiphysis; and thirdly, avascular necrosis within the epiphysis which is a familiar cause of delayed ossification when the vascular supply is compromised in congenital dislocation of the hip.

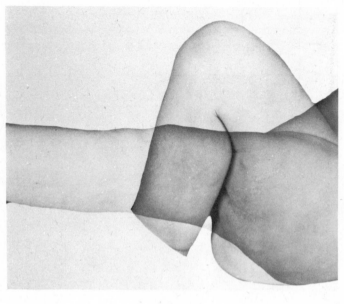

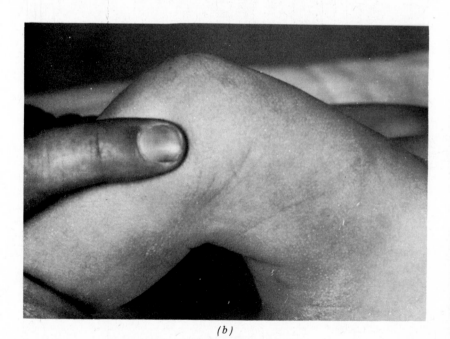

Figure 3.4. Movement is well preserved (a) and the "missing" femoral condyle is palpable (b)

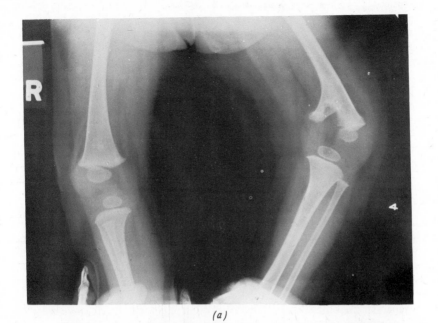

(a)

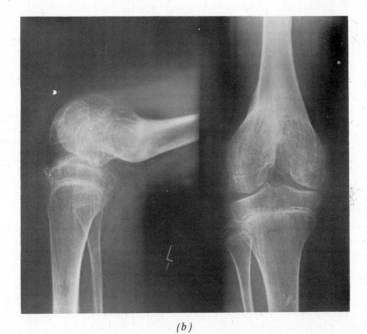

(b)

Figure 3.5. Soon after the acute infection the femoral condyle and growth plate are apparently destroyed (a). The outcome 13 years later (b)

97

Treatment

Management may be discussed in relation to the three phases of the disease, namely, at the time of diagnosis, following the acute illness but before walking begins, and in the late established stage.

(a) *Treatment at the time of diagnosis*

We have three urgent duties to perform. Firstly, we must prescribe antibiotics and general supportive measures; secondly, the hip must be decompressed; and lastly, the hip should be splinted in abduction.

The selection of the most suitable antibiotics before isolation of the invading organism is difficult but, in general, bactericidal drugs are preferable to bacteriostatic. Cloxicillin, supported by some other agent, administered by injection is the usual combination. New, and often more potent, antibiotics are being constantly developed, often with the property of destroying the relatively resistant staphylococcus with greater efficiency. It is prudent, therefore, to seek the advice of a colleague in microbiology at this stage for his help will certainly be needed later in the isolation of the responsible organism and in advising upon its sensitivity to the wide range of alternative antibiotics.

General management may involve transfusion of blood or fluids for dehydration and nutrition if haemolysis or vomiting are prominent. Toxic convulsions or the effects of, for example, associated cerebral or pulmonary infection may dominate the clinical state at any stage so that the help of a paediatrician is essential.

Investigations will, of course, have included blood culture, umbilical and throat swabs, the examination of the haematological values, radiographs and other examinations dictated by the general condition.

In the future we may develop specific methods of substitution for those with immunodeficiency which may favourably modify the degree of destruction locally and the risk of metastatic lesion. For the present, however, fresh, whole blood remains the only measure available to us.

Treatment of the local lesion within the hip is the next priority. The objectives are decompression and drainage together with isolation of the infecting organism. It is often proposed that the first step be aspiration of the hip. This may be justified if the diagnosis is in doubt or the baby's general condition is very poor, but otherwise this manoeuvre represents little more than unwarrantable procrastination (Paterson, 1970). Reluctance to open the hip in a baby derives from the old fear of anaesthesia at this age, an anxiety which advances in neonatal techniques have overtaken. Aspiration, at best, enables us to isolate the infecting agent and instil antibiotics but does little to decompress the hip joint, except briefly, for the puncture will promptly close. Furthermore, the noxious proteolytic pus is unlikely to be completely evacuated for fibrinous adhesions rapidly form pockets within which pus becomes inaccessible (Obletz, 1960).

It is preferable, therefore, to approach the hip directly either posteriorly or anterolaterally between tensor fascia femoris and gluteus medius. The posterior approach is simple and gains access by splitting gluteus maximus in the line of its fibres as in the 'Southern approach' for the insertion of a femoral prosthesis. Nerves are relatively large in babies so the area of the sciatic should be respected.

The short rotators do not obscure the joint capsule which is seen to bulge towards the surgeon. Trial aspiration releases fluid under tension which, in favourable cases, is predominantly blood-tinged and synovial with flakes of fibrin, or, if unfavourable, frank pus. This is preserved for culture. The puncture is enlarged to admit a curved instrument with which to seek and break down loculating adhesions and the nozzle of a Thompson–Walker syringe is introduced for irrigation. The hole should then be further enlarged to ensure that drainage and decompression are maintained when fluid reaccumulates and pressure builds up. The capsular wound remains open but the muscle is loosely closed and the skin sutured.

Our next responsibility is to splint the hip in abduction, not only to replace a dislocation or align a pathological fracture, but also to neutralize any tendency to flexion and adduction deformity which may still predispose to dislocation within the unduly stretched and recently distended capsule. It should also not be forgotten that rest is still an essential element in the treatment of inflammation. Denis Browne's hip harness is ideal for the purpose but an alternative may be made of plaster with a strong posterior slab attached to plaster cuffs around the thighs. This is most conveniently applied with the baby prone with the hips abducted over the end of the table. Both methods leave the wound exposed.

We must now await developments, prescribing antibiotics for at least 6 weeks, and more if indicated, by sedimentation rate and general assessment. Recurrence of fever may indicate a hitherto unsuspected focus elsewhere, so vigilance is necessary. Splinting should certainly be maintained for three months as a measure of rest, and to prevent troublesome deformity.

(b) *Treatment in early childhood*

The decision to explore the hip or withhold operation should if possible be taken at about 1 year of age. This time is chosen because by now the infection will be quiescent and there is a risk in further delay, for walking may displace a pseudarthrosis secondary to a pathological fracture in the femoral neck or, in the event of dislocation or actual capital destruction, cause further upward displacement which adds to the difficulties of repair if operation is performed later. Furthermore, by this age, ossification will usually have advanced into the neck and capital epiphysis enabling us, to some extent, to assess the residual damage. If the area remains translucent we have no such capability and exploration is the only reliable method available to reveal the actual situation and proceed to whatever form of repair seems feasible. A persistent sinus is not usually an inhibiting feature, being rare unless the disease has spread to the femoral shaft.

Operation will, of course, be unnecessary if the acute illness was treated vigorously and promptly and the femoral head has survived within the acetabulum in continuity with the femur. This is, unfortunately, still too rarely seen. When continuity without displacement is present we are more likely to see irregular or delayed ossification of the epiphysis indicating avascular necrosis, which may, however, be compatible with a favourable outcome if it is not associated with partial destruction. When the damage is greater, stiffness is uncommon in spite of ankylosis of the hip, for there is likely to be loss of part of the femoral neck. A mobile pseudarthrosis, with displacement of the femur, then develops and mobility with instability follows. If, however, the head remains within the acetabulum in continuity with the femur, we gain little by protecting the hip during this healing phase and nothing by operating, so observation is the only course. There will be a tendency to develop flexion and adduction deformities, so the mother is encouraged to stretch appropriately. This may be unavailing and surgical correction may be indicated later.

Some of these features may not be apparent at 1 year of age but their implications may be deduced by inference and we may thus be prevented from operating unnecessarily. Beware, however, of a wide 'epiphyseal plate' which may indicate potential instability in an otherwise promising situation.

Exploration of the hip is indicated in the remainder, which, in general, comprise those with displacement. The approach is similar to that described in Chapter 1 for proximal femoral deficiency and, again, it is easier to follow the femoral shaft proximally. Pericapsular adhesions involve the glutei and these must be dissected free of the capsule. On opening the hip a mass of scar tissue may, if damage is severe, disorientate the surgeon, but patient dissection will reveal the anatomical abnormality.

One of four lesions will be found – namely, dislocation, pseudarthrosis alone, pseudarthrosis with hip ankylosis, and total destruction. These will be considered separately (Lloyd-Roberts, 1975).

Dislocation   The head will be superior and intracapsular, but intra-articular adhesions will require division to obtain mobility. In appearance, it will resemble a congenital dislocation which has been manipulated and immobilized with incomplete reduction, i.e. there is variable deformity and the articular cartilage is yellow with patchy pock markings, which are areas of necrosis.

The acetabulum may be difficult to find for it is filled with scar tissue which must be removed before it is fully exposed. Reduction is now not only possible but stable in abduction. The capsule will have been widely opened and repair may be imperfect, so that caution is needed to avoid excessive internal rotation in case the hip dislocates behind. If it seems necessary in the interests of stability, a transfixing Kirschner wire may be used to secure reduction.

The postoperative plaster should be maintained in wide abduction for at least two months and followed by Denis Browne's harness when mobilization begins, for adduction deformity is a constant and continuing hazard. By the same token, varus osteotomy should be avoided. Six months later, full mobilization with daily stretching is advisable (*Figure 3.6*).

Antibiotics should, of course, be prescribed after operation in this and the other operations performed at this age, for the risk of recrudescence of infection is significant especially in immunodeficient children.

The results are, on the whole, disappointing but preferable to those of conservatism. Leg length inequality is corrected and stability restored, but we may expect no more than limited hinge movement to be maintained and even this may decrease as ankylosis develops. There is a marked tendency to the development of adduction and flexion deformity, indicating corrective osteotomy later.

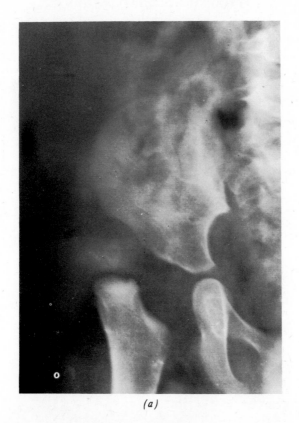

(a)

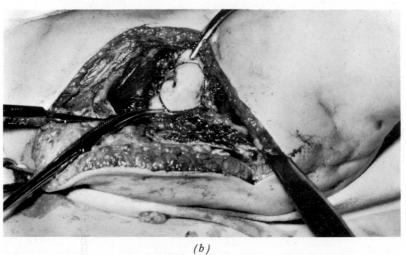

(b)

*Figure 3.6. The pre-operative radiograph (a) shows that the hip is dislocated and the
fate of the capital epiphysis is uncertain. At operation (b) the epiphysis is found to be
intact and relatively normal*

101

Pseudarthrosis This is potentially the most favourable lesion to treat. At operation the mobile area is easily identified. If there is no significant displacement it is probably advisable not to interfere with the pseudarthrosis other than

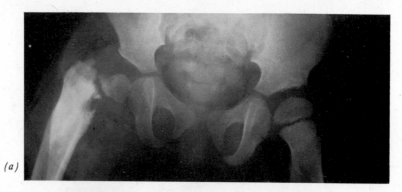

(a)

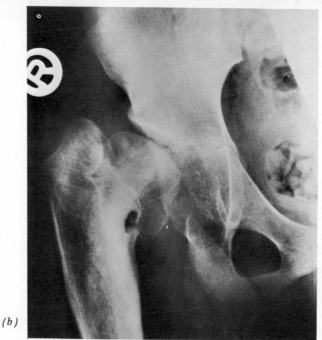

(b)

Figure 3.7. There is a pseudarthrosis in the neck of the femur (a). Following onlay grafting and an abduction displacement osteotomy the pseudarthrosis has united with some deformity and acetabular insufficiency (b)

to onlay cancellous bone which is readily available nearby. An intertrochanteric osteotomy displaced so that the distal fragment lies below the pseudarthrosis and abducted to align the weak area horizontally rather than vertically is now required. Non-union has not caused anxiety (*Figure 3.7*).

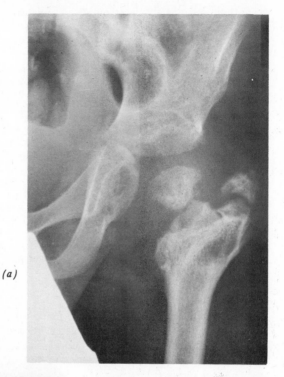

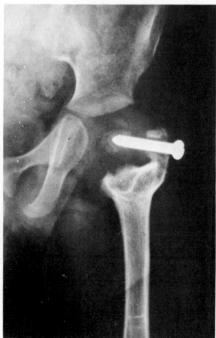

Figure 3.8. A pseudarthrosis separating a relatively normal epiphysis and femoral neck was found on exploring the hip. This was secured by a screw, grafts were applied and an osteotomy performed (a). Eighteen months later these structures are visible and the hip is stable (b)

If there is some displacement, which may be no more than rotation of the epiphysis, it is preferable to secure the epiphyseal fragment with a screw or some other device and prepare a bed for onlay and inlay grafts. An osteotomy should follow as before (*Figure 3.8*).

The results in both the preceding varieties are satisfying for stability is assured, length discrepancy corrected and useful movement retained. The neck rather than the head seems to have been the major target of the original infection and consequently ankylosis has not occurred. It is surprising, therefore, that an unstable and widely displaced pseudarthrosis with a mobile head has not been seen. Should it materialize, I would probably attempt fusion between the trochanter and capital epiphysis with gluteal advancement — an operation which is of proven value in proximal femoral deficiency (*see* page 25).

Some radiological deterioration is to be expected with further growth, taking the form of epiphyseal deformity and acetabular dysplasia. This suggests that the joint has not escaped damage entirely. Movement and growth have been well maintained and secondary deformity avoided.

Abduction osteotomy may also be employed to improve hip stability even when the head is lost but the neck is in contact with the acetabulum (Eyre-Brook, 1960).

Destruction of the head and neck or pseudarthrosis with ankylosis of the hip. These findings may be considered together for they share in common a degree of damage which prevents reconstruction of a mobile hip joint from its component parts. When the epiphysis and neck are destroyed, the trochanteric area will certainly have moved upwards. If there is a pseudarthrosis with ankylosis there will probably be less displacement, but repair of the pseudarthrosis will achieve no more than unsound ankylosis of the hip with a tendency to secondary deformity.

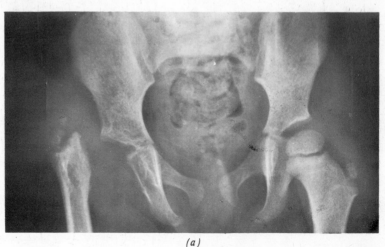

(a)

Figure 3.9. There is destruction of the epiphysis and neck. The trochanter has moved upwards (a)

In the past, I have performed immediate trochanteric—acetabular arthrodesis, accepting the loss of movement and further shortening in the interests of maintaining stability. I now believe that if arthrodesis is chosen it should be deferred until adolescence when overgrowth of the great trochanter may be utilized to overcome some of the shortening.

Trochanteric arthroplasty, however, seems a preferable alternative (Weissman, 1967). The acetabulum is cleared of its contents which, depending upon the variety, will be either dense scar tissue or the surviving epiphysis adherent to it. In either event, there will be some difficulty in establishing the position of

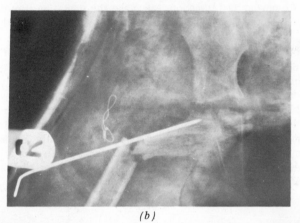

(b)

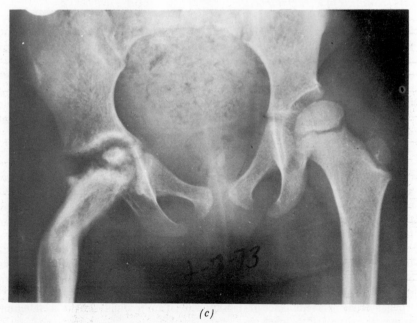

(c)

Figure 3.9. Following trochanteric arthroplasty, gluteal advancement, osteotomy and Kirschner wire fixation (b). The situation one year later (c)

the acetabulum and the correct plane of dissection within it. The glutei having been detached, the great trochanter will be found to be too large to engage the acetabulum deeply. Cartilage should be pared from it until this is possible in the stable position of wide abduction. A Kirschner wire secures the femur to the pelvis and the glutei are advanced as far distally as possible on the femoral shaft.

The position of wide abduction clearly indicates an adduction osteotomy 6 to 8 weeks later if stability is to be maintained in the erect position of walking. The femur lies at a considerable depth and this, together with the difficulty of localizing the new gluteal insertion, can make the operation tiresome. This can be avoided if, at the first operation, a strong wire suture is placed through the femur at the level of intended section and left long so that the surgeon may follow it to the bone. A simple osteotomy is performed to bring the leg to the neutral position. Internal fixation is not necessary providing that the Kirschner wire is retained to be removed at a later date.

This is useful but at best a salvage procedure. Stability is maintained but length is not gained because of the varus angulation and indeed more will be lost during further growth as the capital growth plate has been destroyed and the trochanteric plate is now unlikely to contribute significantly. Some movement, nonetheless, will be achieved and maintained which, with stability, will be of value to the patient. There is a tendency, however, for the osteotomy to straighten with time and this may indicate its revision (*Figure 3.9*).

(c) *Treatment in later childhood*

It has already been indicated that two broad patterns of residual damage are probable in neglected or unsuccessfully treated patients. We may see, on the one hand, a loss of continuity at the femoral neck with marked upward displacement of the trochanter, instability and severe shortening but free mobility. On the other hand, the femur may be in continuity throughout with variable damage to the hip joint and capital growth plate resulting in stability with variable deformity, loss of movement and sometimes moderate shortening. These merit separate discussion.

(1) *Unstable hips*

In early childhood the disability is moderate and compatible with full function despite an unstable hip limp. With time and increasing height and weight the limp becomes more pronounced as the shortening increases and there are complaints of tiredness and aching pain on exertion. Sooner or later the ugliness of the gait will be protested.

The radiograph will reveal wide displacement and proximal lengthening of the trochanteric epiphysis and frequently the femoral head will appear in the acetabulum as a reminder of lost opportunities (*Figure 3.10*). The hemi-pelvis may be smaller than its fellow. There is sometimes overgrowth of the lesser trochanter giving a semblance of stability when it approximates to the acetabulum, as may the stump of the neck.

Treatment alternatives are limited. To accept the situation is to settle for a state which is cosmetically unacceptable to most and uncomfortable in some.

Total hip replacement has not yet achieved that degree of refinement to make it a subject for consideration, though it may be considered in later life to replace an arthrodesis performed at this stage.

Notwithstanding its disadvantages, arthrodesis requires serious consideration, even in girls in spite of the well-known problems that this generates for them because they are the more likely to complain of a cosmetic disability. The advantages are restoration of stability, neutralization of the lurching gait and relief of discomfort if this is present. There will, furthermore, be some reduction in the true shortening for, as already mentioned, there is overgrowth of the great

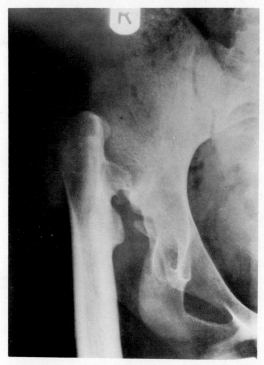

Figure 3.10. The late effects of an untreated hip. The epiphysis and part of the neck are now visible

trochanter which may be harnessed to help. The element due to upward displacement is also reduced. In this connection it is important to realize that the distance between the tip of the trochanter and the lateral malleolus may be almost equal to that on the other side.

It is evident that a decision to perform an arthrodesis must be taken only after careful consideration and discussion with the patient. It has already been mentioned that arthrodesis should be avoided in early childhood in spite of the probability of success at that time. Delaying operation allows the trochanter to grow, maintains mobility in early childhood, and permits full discussion with the patient at an age (usually about 15 years) when he can express his views. The onset of aching pain will simplify the decision but this is far from constant. It is also sometimes helpful to mimic the loss of movement by using a short hip spica. In general, however, there is no substitute for explanation and discussion, especially with the girls. Boys and girls may be told about the possibility of replacement in the future and the boys encouraged by the good functional results of arthrodesis in the absence of involvement of other joints.

The recommended (if not the only possible) technique is acetabulo-trochanteric compression arthrodesis. The hip is approached from the lateral side using either Gibson's incision or preferably a goblet incision. The glutei are detached with a

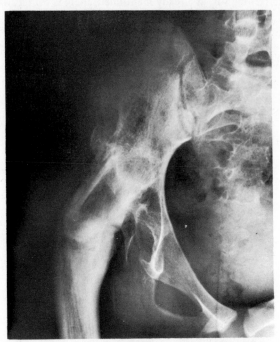

Figure 3.11. The result of two-stage compression
arthrodesis

sliver of bone and the trochanter decorticated on its lateral, anterior and posterior surfaces. The medial surface and tip are denuded of soft tissue only to maintain stability and length. The acetabulum is cleared of soft tissue and reamed in such a way that a gallery is produced within and upwards from the lip. The remaining articular cartilage is excised and the trochanter slipped into the gallery with the leg abducted to about 60°, which produces both compression and stability. It may sometimes be necessary to shorten the trochanter slightly in order to pass it deep to the acetabular lip. Locally-available cancellous bone is packed into the remaining unfilled acetabulum and the glutei secured to the femoral shaft at a lower level to increase stability. Plaster is applied in this position and maintained for two months when an osteotomy is performed to bring the leg to the neutral position and plastered thus. Union of both is usually sound 4 months later. The osteotomy is simplified if a wire marker is inserted at the first stage as previously described (see page 106).

In my experience the early results of arthrodesis are rewarding and preferred by the patient to the pre-existing situation (Bryson, 1948). The boys are functionally good and the girls, if walking slowly, have an almost imperceptible limp. Angulation of the osteotomy site will tend to diminish and encourage speculation about replacement in the future (*Figure 3.11*).

(2) *Stable hips*   The variability of the initial damage causing less than bone loss or dislocation will be reflected in the variability of the outcome in relation to pain, movement and shortening. Some of these features will be further discussed.

Diagnosis may be difficult when there is no reliable history of neonatal illness specifically affecting the hip or of a septicaemic illness responding rapidly to antibiotics. The radiographic signs will be those of any quiescent arthritis with, perhaps, coxa magna, deformity of the head, acetabular deficiency, loss of joint space and possibly subluxation or shortening of the neck and undue prominence of the trochanter if the growth plate is affected. The signs of variable loss of movement, deformity and shortening will, in some, be associated with limp if growth is affected, and with pain if capital ischaemia complicates the situation.

Treatment will be orientated towards the relief of symptoms and the methods are similar to those indicated when pyogenic arthritis affects the older child (*see* page 113). The hip joint is not amenable to repair but diagnostic biopsy may, even today, be necessary to exclude tuberculosis or perhaps juvenile rheumatoid arthritis though monarticular hip involvement is very unusual.

It is most important to appreciate two complementary observations. Firstly, there is a tendency for movement to increase with time with, in consequence, a reduction in the degree of deformity to an acceptable level. Secondly, the earlier we perform a corrective osteotomy the more probable is recurrence of deformity during further growth. It is better, therefore, to delay such an operation for as long as limited movement coupled with deformity permit reasonable function.

Arthrodesis is most likely to be required when ischaemia has caused pain due to capital collapse with unsound ankylosis in deformity. Intertrochanteric osteotomy alone may result in hip fusion, but failure will almost certainly be followed by recurring deformity so that sound hip fusion is desirable. Even then, further mild deformity may develop in the younger children, so delay is again advocated when this is possible. Girls are again at a disadvantage but the alternative of excisional arthroplasty is also undesirable.

A satisfactory technique retains the hip joint in the position of deformity which is maintained by inlay corticocancellous grafts applied in front and above with cancellous chips impacted wherever a small gap may be developed between head and acetabulum. Internal fixation will only be necessary if significant movement is still possible and should be limited to 2 Knowle's pins which penetrate the inner pelvic wall. An osteotomy with medial displacement is then performed to correct deformity and a plaster applied in the desired position (Apley and Denham, 1955). Following union there remains the possibility of hip replacement in later life under more favourable conditions than those following trochanteric fusion.

Two further possibilities merit discussion. Inequality of leg length is better treated by contralateral shortening if the adult height permits. Femoral leg-lengthening introduces the hazard not only of further damage to a mobile hip by upward compression but also of damage to the hitherto normal knee by downward compression — a risk which persists even when the hip is fused. Gluteal insufficiency due to femoral-neck shortening and trochanteric overgrowth is sometimes seen in Perthes' disease and congenital dislocation and is alleviated by advancing the gluteal attachment distally with the trochanter (*see* page 79). A similar operation has been equally satisfactory in one patient with quiescent pyogenic arthritis.

It should not be assumed from the descriptions of the residual problems and their management that these are acceptable or justifiable. Aggressive and early primary treatment should result in a high incidence of complete recovery or at least only minor damage predisposing to osteoarthritis in later life (Watkins, Samilson and Winters, 1956; Paterson, 1970).

PYOGENIC ARTHRITIS IN THE OLDER CHILD

In contrast to neonatal disease, there are relatively few features of specific importance to the hip joint when the presentation is late. The bacterial spectrum is similar, but portals of entry are inevitably different — i.e. throat and skin sepsis replacing the umbilicus and injection sites. The chondrolytic effect of pus is, of course, lessened as bone replaces cartilage. We have not studied immunological factors in disease arising in this age group.

Differential diagnosis may be difficult in spite of the virtual disappearance of rheumatic fever and tuberculosis, which, in this situation sometimes presents in unexpectedly acute form. Juvenile rheumatoid arthritis should not cause confusion if it is remembered that the age of highest incidence is between 2 and 5 years of age and that monarticular hip involvement is rare.

Considerable difficulty may arise in some patients with unusually severe non-specific synovitis with fever, extreme hip irritability and even leucocytosis with a raised sedimentation rate. There seems to be a fault in their response to infection elsewhere, (which is usually upper respiratory), with hypersensitivity secondary to auto-immunity. These episodes may be repeated, which is an aid to diagnosis. Aspiration of the hip is indicated but upon two occasions we have elected to explore the joint because of continuing uncertainty.

Lastly, subacute periarticular osteomyelitis with an irritable hip and an area of translucency within the femoral neck or trochanteric area, haemarthrosis in bleeding diseases, capital necrosis of sickling anaemia, and Gaucher's disease and severe arthralgia in the specific fevers, may all contribute to the problem. A bone-scan or estimation of the staphylococcal titres may be valuable in subacute infection.

It is generally assumed that organisms attack the joint either directly via the synovial membrane or secondarily from a focus of osteomyelitis within the joint capsule at the level of the capital metaphysis or very occasionally from the acetabular side. There is sometimes dispute on this issue reminiscent of similar debates during the tuberculosis era — and it is equally nebulous, for the outcome and management are the same for both.

It is my belief that a primary bone focus is the predominant site of onset but that this focus is not necessarily cervical and intracapsular; more commonly it affects the trochanteric area at the attachment of, or distal to, the joint capsule (Kemp and Lloyd-Roberts, 1974).

This concept introduces a further dimension into our notions of the mechanism by which the joint is damaged and thereby influences our management.

The mechanism of joint damage

The conventional belief that synovial or intracapsular metaphyseal infection damages the hip by a combination of direct bacterial attack and synovial pannus aided by raised intra-articular tension and later by the chondrolytic effect of pus, is valid so far as some varieties are concerned. It does not, however, fully explain the mechanism when infection arises in the trochanteric region.

It is necessary to describe the differences for I believe that primary trochanteric infection is commoner than the intra-articular, so that in most we have an opportunity to prevent infection reaching the joint rather than having to treat intra-articular infection arising *de novo*. There are two stages in the development of the untreated disease. Firstly, we have the vascular component and, secondly, the infective. The arterial anastomosis from which the vessels supplying the epiphysis arise, surrounds the trochanteric area so that infection therein is likely to be followed by thrombosis of these vessels which compromise the epiphyseal supply. Sympathetic joint effusions are commonplace in association with extra-capsular metaphyseal lesions and are especially familiar around the knee where they are immediately apparent. Such an effusion within the hip is occult but nonetheless arises. The integrity of the arterial and venous circulation is again at risk if intra-articular pressure increases, for these vessels are particularly vulnerable at the zone of synovial reflection onto the neck. The effects will be apparent after a latent period (*see Figure 3.14*).

Should infection now spread proximally to enter the joint cavity, the invaders encounter ideal circumstances for producing the greatest possible damage, i.e. tissues devitalized by ischaemia together with deep tension. Ischaemia and infection now combine to inflict severe damage upon the joint with great rapidity.

We can, therefore, identify three sequential phases of the disease in the untreated patient: firstly, extracapsular osteomyelitis; secondly, osteomyelitis with ischaemic capital necrosis; and, lastly, osteomyelitis, ischaemic necrosis and suppurative arthritis.

The management

(a) *Acute pyogenic arthritis*

The preliminary steps are similar to those employed in neonatal disease and include a search for a primary focus on the skin or throat and the taking of a swab, blood culture, basic haematological assay, antibiotics, rest with traction, and analgesics for the relief of pain. Careful examination of the trochanteric area is essential and scrutiny of the radiograph is concentrated here.

The urgency of intervention is as great as in neonatal disease but the methods are different. If trochanteric osteomyelitis is suspected, the area is approached between gluteus medius and the tensor fascia femoris. On lifting vastus lateralis, the capsule comes into view and is likely to be bulging. Following aspiration for culture, the capsule is opened and fluid under tension released. The capsular decompression is enlarged by partial excision to prevent premature closure and exploratory drill holes are made in the trochanteric area for drainage and decompression of the bone and the wound is closed.

If, however, the disease is regarded as primarily intra-articular, aspiration and instillation of antibiotics may be sufficient and indeed is an advisable first step if, as is so often the case, the diagnosis is in doubt. This may be followed by drainage through the posterior approach if aspiration having confirmed the diagnosis seems inadequate, of if the symptoms and signs do not resolve rapidly. If indicated, this must not be delayed for Paterson (1970) has shown that drainage with skin closure has been followed by near perfect results providing that it is performed within 5 days of the onset.

In either event the postoperative regime is the same: traction until irritability disappears, followed by crutch-walking and antibiotics for at least the traditional period of 6 weeks.

(b) *The later stages of the disease*

The outcome will be variable depending upon such factors as virulence, resistance and the vigour and timing of treatment. At best the hip is normal, though there may be coxa magna (*Figure 3.12*). At worst the head is destroyed and the subluxated femoral neck, displaying the stigmata of chronic osteomyelitis, abuts upon the pelvis.

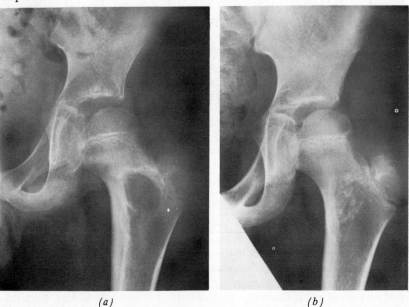

(a)   (b)

Figure 3.12. Following prompt and aggressive treatment the hip joint is preserved. Note the residual bone cavity following curettage and the slight extrusion of the femoral head (a). One year later healing is satisfactory with some degree of coxa magna (b)

Our immediate concern revolves around ischaemia of the femoral head which, as previously mentioned, may be septic or aseptic. If ischaemia is complicated by spreading infection, this is apparent within 2 to 3 weeks. The head retains its normal shape but becomes opaque in comparison with the surrounding bone. The

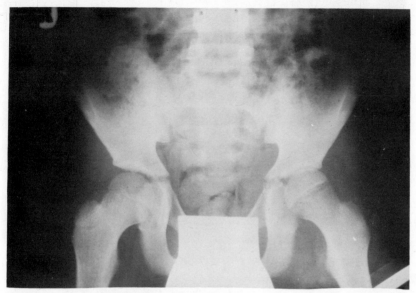

Figure 3.13. (a) Soon after the infection was brought under control, the femoral head is normal but the joint space is reduced

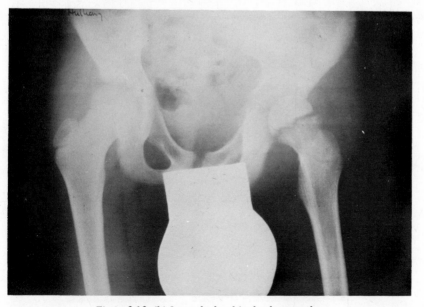

Figure 3.13. (b) Later the head is clearly avascular

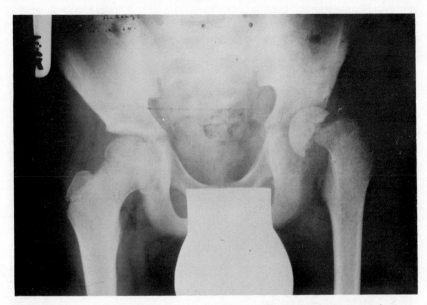

Figure 3.13. (c) The head has separated as a sequestrum and was removed

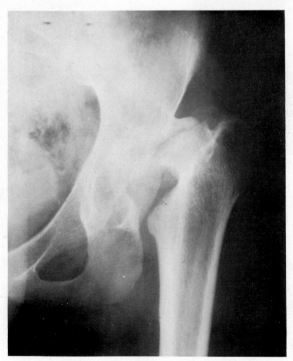

Figure 3.13. (d) The final outcome

114

head then separates at the epiphyseal plate, the neck moves upwards and the leg adducts. The head is now a sequestrum and, if infection with or without a sinus persists, it must be removed (*Figure 3.13*). Some, of course, will be less florid, in which case some degree of prevarication is possible. The management is similar to that outlined for the late effects of neonatal arthritis (*see* page 107).

Aseptic necrosis without infection will take longer to declare itself and may not be suspected radiologically for between 6 to 8 weeks (*Figure 3.14*). Clinically, however, irritability of the hip will persist as a warning sign. Ischaemia may be segmental or total; the former resembles Perthes' disease in its subsequent course, but the latter behaves differently. It is not analagous to whole-head Perthes' disease (Catterall Group 4; *see* page 129), for limitation of movement amounting to partial ankylosis and deformity frequently follow. If mobility is well maintained, it would seem reasonable to proceed as though dealing with Perthes' disease. If not, corrective osteotomy is our recourse.

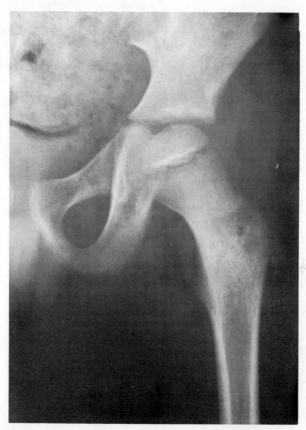

(a)

Figure 3.14. Shortly after the acute infection has been controlled, the hip appears to have escaped damage (a)

(b)(i)

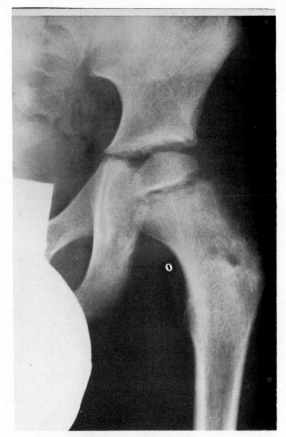

(b)(ii)

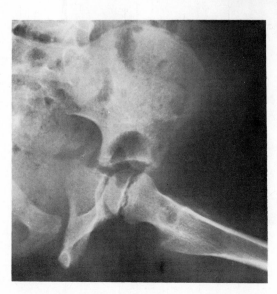

Figure 3.14. Two months later a residual bone cavity is visible and the epiphysis is becoming dense with a more translucent area in front (b)

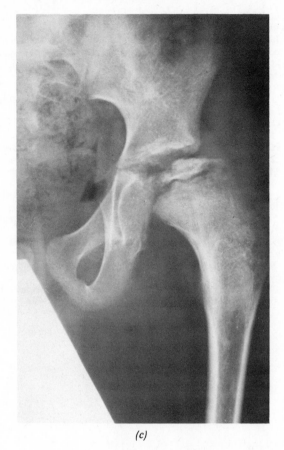

(c)

Figure 3.14. Eight months later epiphyseal necrosis
is evident (c)

Within the limits of these extremes, we see hips with varying degrees of residual damage whose management must be adapted to the clinical problem. The observations already made upon the late treatment of stable hips following neonatal arthritis apply equally to this group (*see* page 107).

REFERENCES

Apley, A. G. and Denham, R. A. (1955). Osteotomy as an aid to arthrodesis of the hip. *J. Bone Jt Surg.* **37B**, 185

Brown, I. (1975). A study of the 'capsular' shadow in disorders of the hip in children. *J. Bone Jt Surg.* **57B**, 175

Bryson, A. F. (1948). Treatment of pathological dislocation of the hip joint after suppurative arthritis in infants. *J. Bone Jt Surg.* **30B**, 449

Chacha, P. B. (1971). Suppurative arthritis of the hip joint in infancy. A persistent diagnostic problem and possible complication of femoral veni-puncture. *J. Bone Jt Surg.* **53A**, 538

REFERENCES

Eyre-Brook, A. L. (1960). Septic arthritis of the hip and osteomyelitis of the upper end of the femur in infants. *J. Bone Jt Surg.* **42B,** 11

Kemp, H. and Lloyd-Roberts, G. C. (1974). Avascular necrosis of the capital epiphysis following osteomyelitis of the proximal femoral metaphysis. *J. Bone Jt Surg.* **56B,** 688

Kuo, K. N., Lloyd-Roberts, G. C., Orme, I. M. and Soothill, J. F. (1975). Immunodeficiency and infantile bone and joint infection. *Archs Dis. Childh.* **50,** 51

Lack, C. H. (1959). Chondrolysis in arthritis. *J. Bone Jt Surg.* **41B,** 384

Lloyd-Roberts, G. C. (1960). Suppurative arthritis of infancy. Some observations upon prognosis and management. *J. Bone Jt Surg.* **42B,** 706

Lloyd-Roberts, G. C. (1975). Some aspects of orthopaedic surgery in childhood. *Ann. R. Coll. Surg.* **57,** 25

Obletz, B. E. (1960). Acute suppurative arthritis of the hip in the neonatal period. *J. Bone Jt Surg.* **42A,** 23

Paterson, D. C. (1970). Acute suppurative arthritis in infancy and childhood. *J. Bone Jt Surg.* **52B,** 474

Phemister, D. B. (1924). Changes in the articular surfaces in tuberculosis and in pyogenic infections of joints. *Am. J. Roentg.* **12,** 1

Phemister, D. B. (1924). The effect of pressure on articular surfaces in pyogenic and tuberculous arthritis and its bearing on treatment. *Ann. Surg.* **80,** 481

Trueta, J. (1959). The three types of acute haematogenous osteomyelitis. A clinical and vascular study. *J. Bone Jt Surg.* **41B,** 671

Watkins, M. B., Samilson, R. L., and D. M. Winters (1956). Acute suppurative arthritis. *J. Bone Jt Surg.* **38A,** 1313

Weissman, S. L. (1967). Transplantation of the trochanteric epiphysis into the acetabulum after septic arthritis of the hip. Report of a case. *J. Bone Jt Surg.* **49A,** 1647

4

Perthes' Disease–Part I
Pathogenesis, Classification and Treatment

G. C. Lloyd- Roberts

During recent years there has been a renewal of effort directed towards a better understanding of the nature of Perthes' disease. The emphasis has been on the morbid anatomy, aetiology (including genetics), experimental methods of simulation and classification in relation to prognosis. The ultimate purpose of these investigations was, of course, to help us to rationalize our methods of treatment which have consequently undergone radical changes.

I do not propose to outline the well-known history of the identification of the disease and the early debates concerning its management, nor will I describe in detail the clinical features and the evolution of the radiological sequence for these are familiar or readily available. I shall concentrate, therefore, upon the topics mentioned above with special emphasis upon those aspects which seem to be related to contemporary attitudes to treatment, which in turn will be discussed in some detail.

PATHOLOGY OF PERTHES' DISEASE

Morbid anatomy

The opportunity to examine an intact hip joint is, in the nature of things, rarely offered. When it has been offered we find that most reports are disappointing for they have neglected to correlate the macroscopic and microscopic features with the radiographic features using microradiography. An exception is the report by McKibbin and Ralis (1974) which will be my main reference point. More such carefully studied specimens are needed if we are to interpret radiographs — which are our only readily available means of assay — correctly.

Descriptions of the intact epiphysis have in common the observation that the anterosuperior segment is flattened and that there is a concave depression medial to this (*Figure 4.1*). Observations on the living are even more scanty but from the evidence of one patient I can confirm this and add that the articular cartilage, although yellow, did not yield to direct pressure in the manner of a ping-pong ball. The natural history is prolonged and during this time the epiphysis may undergo considerable modifications in contour so that observations upon one, or even a few, specimens cannot be expected to cover the whole spectrum of

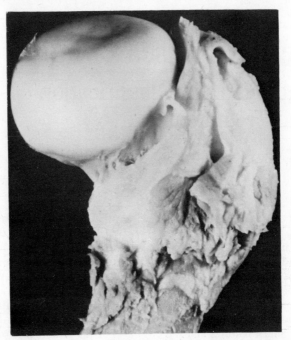

Figure 4.1. The appearance of the head from a patient with Perthes' disease showing the central depression (Reproduced from McKibbin and Rallis (1974) by permission)

change. Furthermore, we lack precise descriptions of gross and, to some extent, microscopic changes in the acetabulum, growth plate, metaphysis and femoral neck.

The microscopic appearances within the epiphysis are those of segmental necrosis undergoing revascularization, but here again we are at a disadvantage for one specimen, *Figure 4.2*, only discloses the changes at one stage in one patient suffering from one pattern of a disease of variable intensity. Nonetheless there is general agreement that areas of normal bone alternate with areas of necrosis undergoing osteoclastic absorption and replacement by granulation and, later, fibrous tissue. Elsewhere, there is active osteoblastic activity with new bone laid down on the surface of dead trabeculae. Some areas are hyperaemic and some avascular. There is debate as to whether compression stress fractures are responsible for some of the changes (Harrison, 1976) or whether these appearances represent a disproportion between absorption and new bone formation involving one trabecula. This has some relevance to treatment for, if fractures are commonplace, protection from weight-bearing would seem to be indicated (McKibbin, 1975).

We can now explain three of the radiographic signs for, in McKibbin and Ralis' specimen, the microscopic fields were correlated by microradiography. Increased opacity represents new bone ensheathing dead trabeculae and translucency areas of absorption and fibrous replacement. Widening of the joint space is commonly seen and is a valuable aid to diagnosis. Ischaemia affects the germinal bone-forming cells in the epiphysis so that ossification does not spread from the bony nucleus towards the periphery. At the same time, there is some cartilage proliferation in the surface layers nourished by synovial fluid. Thus, there is both a relative and absolute increase in the thickness of the cartilage and, thus also, of the joint space.

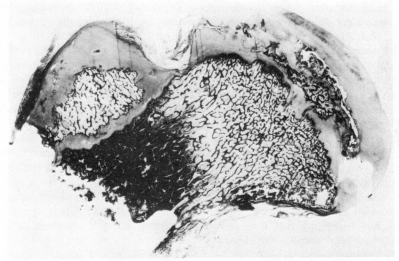

Figure 4.2. Microradiograph of Figure 4.1. showing apparent thickening of the articular cartilage with necrotic bone below. Note the penetration of the growth plate (Reproduced from McKibbin and Ralis (1974) by permission)

When ischaemia is severe and involves the greater part of the head, we sometimes see premature closure of the growth plate. This is not surprising for the germinal cells being nourished from the epiphyseal side become inactive. Furthermore, metaphyseal vessels may cross the plate to provide a collateral circulation to the ischaemic nucleus and complete the process.

Premature closure is followed by identifiable changes in the clinical radiograph. The neck shortens (the leg also) and widens, due perhaps to collateral hyperaemia of its periosteum or as a biomechanical response to the flattening and widening of the head which commonly develops. There is overgrowth of the trochanteric epiphysis so that the tip is displaced proximally. In summation there may be a bony block to abduction and gluteal insufficiency (Robichon *et al.*, 1974).

Areas of translucency are frequently seen within the metaphysis — the so-called cysts. They usually lie in relation to dense areas (active bone-forming zones) in the epiphysis. The pathogenesis is unknown but, on occasion, they are large and so unlikely to represent erosion around fractures through the epiphyseal plate. Continuing growth-plate activity without ossification in the affected area is a possibility when the cysts are small but again they cannot account for the larger cysts unless some process causes decalcification in the surrounding bone of the neck (Ponseti, 1956).

Irregularity within the subchondral bone of the acetabulum is sometimes seen in radiographs but we have no microscopic correlation. It is possible that these changes signify the rearrangements necessary when the acetabulum adapts its shape to that of a deformed head to bring about a state of 'congruous incongruity' of the hip joint (see later).

Lastly, we must consider the synovial membrane and capsule. Unfortunately the autopsy studies pay scant attention to the soft tissues. It is generally assumed that there is chronic synovitis with capsular thickening and it has been suggested that secondary obliterative vascular changes may modify the quality of synovial fluid, thus affecting the nutrition of articular cartilage (Ferguson and Howarth, 1934; Hipp, 1962). Bulging of a thickened capsule, due allegedly to a combination of chronic synovitis and excess fluid, is often described as one of the characteristic radiological signs. This 'capsular line' is, however, an artefact as Brown (1975) working in this hospital has recently shown. The line represents an intermuscular plane and its position is dependent upon that of the hip joint.

Nonetheless, chronic synovitis is a probable feature and, unless we assume that it is present, it is difficult to account for lateral extrusion of the femoral head away from the acetabulum. This extrusion is evident as an increase in the gap between the medial and inferior corner of the metaphysis and the teardrop shadow and it is quite distinct from the widening of the joint space above this, which is due to increased thickness of unossified cartilage. Furthermore, this medial gap is not reduced when the hip is adducted and it is increased in abduction suggesting that it is caused by some translucent structure in this area, which is presumably soft tissue.

Pathogenesis

We may assume from autopsy and biopsy studies that the essential lesion is an infarct of the capital epiphysis and that the other observed changes in the surrounds are secondary to this.

Having accepted this proposition, we must attempt to answer some awkward questions. Why and how does the infarct occur? Why does healing by osteoblastic substitution take so long? Why is the outcome usually so favourable, compared with capital ischaemia due to injury which frequently in a child ends in ankylosis.

Explanations other than ischaemia are sometimes offered varying from the original suspicion of underlying infection to the recent concept of delay in skeletal development affecting the capital epiphysis and exposing it to compression fracture as the child gains in weight (Harrison, 1976). Nevertheless, on the evidence at present available, we must still regard the basic lesion as ischaemia due to epiphyseal artery occlusion.

Attempts to elucidate the cause and nature of this occlusion by clinical and laboratory research have attracted many workers in recent years and some of their relevant observations will be considered below.

(a) *Clinical research*

We must consider whether there is a predisposition to Perthes' disease in some children as in some animals. For example, the poodle is vulnerable, the beagle immune. So we must look first at the genetic evidence. A definite predisposition is not discernible for monozygotic twins have been reported as discordant, but there is a higher than expected familial incidence (Fisher, 1972). Catterall, Lloyd-Roberts and Wynne-Davies (1971), however, found a significant relationship between congenital abnormalities of the genito-urinary system and inguinal region and Perthes' disease and postulated that if there was some associated vascular anomaly around the hip the epiphyseal circulation might be more precarious than usual. The vascular arrangements of immune and vulnerable dogs differ and it is conceivable that humans share this variability.

Investigations directed towards growth and development in these children have disclosed a high incidence of skeletal maturation-delay and short stature (Goff, 1954; Fisher, 1972; Harrison, Turner and Jacobs, 1976), which again stimulates speculation about the nature of the disease. May it be a local manifestation of a widespread disorder of bone growth which is the essential predisposing influence?

The relationship between transient synovitis and Perthes' disease has been repeatedly investigated but no significant association has been found. This is disappointing because it would have supported the concept of vascular occlusion by articular tamponade (Kemp, 1973).

Vascular patterns have been studied by intra-osseous venography and by the use of isotopes. Venography shows a variation in venous drainage in the early stages in which less blood than normal passes through the local hip-joint veins and more into the diaphysis, which makes us think again of the possible influence of tamponade (Suramo *et al.*, 1974).

Morley (1975) has investigated femoral-head activity by estimating quantitatively the uptake of ^{99}mTc polyphosphate and more recently technetium phosphonate. This work is in a preliminary stage but some interesting observations have already been made. The epiphyseal uptake expressed as a ratio of the uptake at a constant point in the femoral shaft indicates abnormally low levels in the early stages of the disease, but this increases as the disease evolves. So far there has been neither a late fall, which would support the theory of multiple infarction, nor correlation with 'necrotic' areas seen on the radiograph though, in some, increased activity was associated with changes in the femoral neck. Epiphyseal uptake was reduced and remained low for about 6 months following femoral osteotomy. In one patient the diagnosis of Perthes' disease was made by scanning 2 months before there was radiological evidence. This investigation seems to show promise and is continuing.

Lastly, classification, based upon radiological signs correlated with the known microscopic features of density and translucency, helps us to appreciate the extent and situation of the infarct and relate this to prognosis. This aspect will be considered later.

(b) *Laboratory research*

Animal experiments which produce total infarction of the epiphysis do not, as already mentioned, reproduce a model comparable with Perthes' disease as seen in man. Great interest has therefore been aroused by the notion of multiple infarction (Sanchis, Zahir, and Freeman, 1973). A single infarct is followed by rapid healing without deformity whereas, if the insult is repeated in a few weeks, there is both delay in healing and distortion – a situation analogous to that found in the naturally occurring disease. Further support for this theory is found in McKibbin and Ralis' specimen in which the evidence for a double infarct was persuasive (*Figure 4.3*). Some bone showed signs of earlier appositional new bone on dead trabeculae pre-dating a more recent episode of infarction

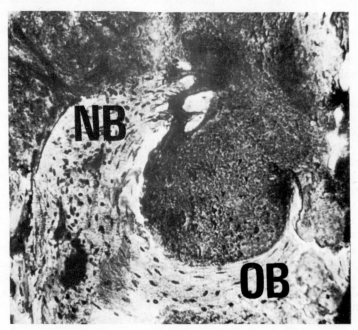

Figure 4.3. There is evidence of multiple infarction with old bone (OB) *and new bone* (NB) *co-existing* (Reproduced from McKibbin and Ralis (1974) by permission)

which, in turn, affected this appositional bone. Furthermore recurrent Perthes' disease has been described (Kemp and Baijens, 1971). Residual osteochondritis is not uncommon (Ratliff, 1967b; Kamhi and MacEwen, 1975), implying that one final infarct may have been irreparable.

Further ingenious experiments (Spivey and Park, 1973) using glass microemboli also produce variable degrees of ischaemia and changes resembling human disease. The results suggest that in some respects the epiphyseal and metaphyseal effects are independent, being related to the site of vascular occlusion. It is possible that large metaphyseal cysts are a reflection of a local nutrient artery occlusion rather than secondary to epiphyseal ischaemia.

The mechanism of vascular insufficiency has been studied by Kemp (1973) in a series of elegant experiments in which he raised the intra-articular pressure (tamponade) in susceptible and immune dogs. In the susceptible animals (poodles) the extra-osseous course of the epiphyseal artery was longer than in the immune (beagles). Only the poodles suffered epiphyseal ischaemia which was in all respects similar to Perthes' disease occurring naturally in this species. Pressures as low as 40 mmHg were sufficient, suggesting that venous occlusion alone might be responsible, thus correlating well with the observations made during intra-osseous venography previously mentioned. Recurrent synovitis could then explain recurrent infarction if a correlation between synovitis and Perthes' disease could be demonstrated; this has not been possible at a clinical level.

Lastly, in investigating the mechanism of deformation, Salter (1966) has used the infarcted epiphyses of pigs thereby producing an excellent experimental model. He points out that deformity is due to the effect of abnormal pressure upon the new woven bone of repair which, for a time, is in a state of 'biological plasticity'. This gives powerful experimental support to the concept of treatment by containment (*see later*), for protection from abnormal stress is assured only when the head is congruous with the acetabulum. More recently, he has demon-strated that collapse can cause secondary infarction and still greater deformation.

THE EVOLUTION OF MODERN CONCEPTS OF CLASSIFICATION AND TREATMENT IN PERTHES' DISEASE

Since Perthes' disease was first identified as an entity (pseudocoxalgia) distinct from tuberculosis of the hip, the object of treatment has been the prevention of residual deformity. Opinions have varied between the nihilistic, which assumed that deformity was predestined from the first and uninfluenced by treatment, and the belief that rest in recumbency, prolonged and enforced, would prevent this from happening.

This uncertainty is not surprising for it is a feature of natural evolution that about half of our patients (59 per cent) will heal without significant deformity (Catterall, 1971) (Table 4.1). Although many of those with residual deformity

TABLE 4.I

The overall results of untreated Perthes' disease divided into groups. 59 per cent heal without significant deformity. (Reproduced from Catterall (1971) by permission)

	Good	Fair	Poor
Group 1	27	1	0
Group 2	23	6	2
Group 3	4	7	11
Group 4	0	4	10
	54(59%)	18	23

have a remarkably good clinical outcome (Ratliff, 1967), Helbo (1953) has related osteoarthritis to the degree of this deformity. In a disease so variable in its presentation and consequence, it is still difficult for us to assess the use-fulness or otherwise of any form of treatment let alone the alternative methods that have been employed. Clearly, the results are likely to depend more upon the nature of the sample treated than the method used. In theory it would be possible by chance to achieve 100 per cent good results or 100 per cent bad results by almost any means if the patients treated in each series were representative of good or bad prognosis groups exclusively. The implication is that overall results of any mode of treatment which ignore this fact or neglect to use controls are valueless. Such presentations are responsible for much of the confusion that has arisen.

Even when controls are used but the index patients selected on the basis of criteria which are themselves inaccurate or incomplete, the comparison may lead to misleading conclusions.

We have ourselves twice been guilty of arriving at fallacious conclusions because we used parameters of assessment which were incomplete. Evans and Lloyd-Roberts (1958) compared a combined in-patient (axial traction) and out-patient (caliper) regime with out-patient management alone using a Snyder sling. Excluding girls, the criteria of assessment were the age of onset and the stage of the disease. It was concluded that there was no difference in outcome between the two methods (Table 4.II). Later Murley and Lloyd-Roberts (1962)

TABLE 4.II

A comparison of the results of two methods of conservative treatment not using the containment principle: (a) the clinical material; (b) the results. (Reproduced by permission from Evans and Lloyd-Roberts (1958))

(a)

	In-patient	Out-patient
Number of cases	24	24
Stage:		
Early	12	12
Late	12	12
Treatment:		
Bed rest and traction	10 months	1 week
Caliper	15 months	—
Snyder sling	—	21 months
Total	25 months	21 months
Follow-up:		
Average	6.75 years	4.75 years
Shortest	2.75 years	3.25 years

(b)

Method of treatment	Result Good	Intermediate	Bad
In-patient	15	5	4
Out-patient	14	4	6

used the same criteria and controls to assess untreated hips. The benefits of treatment were so marginal that we doubted whether treatment was justified. The fallacy was due to assuming that treatment by axial traction, caliper and Snyder sling had an influence on the natural history. We now know that they probably do not, and, if this is true, we were comparing like with like and not surprisingly found the results to be similar. Put otherwise we may say that we were comparing one useless method with another.

Nevertheless, Murley made the important observation that some patients with involvement of the whole head seemed to derive some benefit from protection from weight-bearing – a point which was obscured by the similarity of the overall results. It was known at that time that, when only the anterior segment of the head was affected, the prognosis was good (O'Garra, 1959) and it was also assumed that some had already deformed when treatment began and were therefore unlikely to benefit. In spite of this, some hips not included in the above categories had a better outcome when not treated than when treated.

The direction of further investigation was now apparent and Catterall studied in greater detail the radiological signs upon which the prognosis could be forecast in the early stages and, in 1971, he published his now well-known classification. In a survey of untreated patients he described four groups based on the degree of radiological involvement of the capital epiphysis and underlying metaphysis. Group 1 corresponded to O'Garra's half-head variety (*Figure 4.4*). Group 2 and 3 had increasing involvement and 'sequestrum' formation and in Group 4, the whole epiphysis was affected (*Figure 4.5*). The prognosis was proportional to the degree of radiological involvement. Age of onset was a significant factor within the groups and girls, having a tendency towards the more severe varieties, had a worse prognosis than boys.

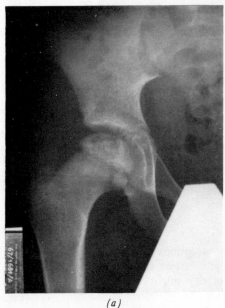

(a)

Figure 4.4. See caption on p. 128

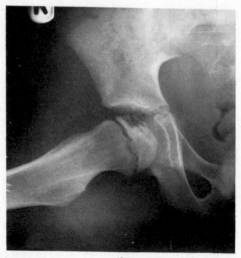

(b)

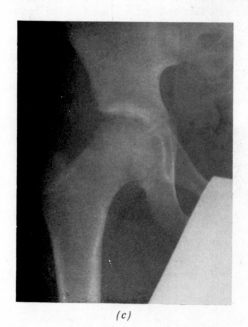

Figure 4.4. Group 1 Perthes' disease (Catterall classification). Rather less than half the head is involved and healing is good without treatment. (Reproduced from Lloyd-Roberts, Orthopaedics in Infancy and Childhood, 1971)

(c)

There were some exceptions to this orderly pattern of evolution, particularly in Groups 2 and 3, and further study identified certain radiological signs which indicated that deformity might occur regardless of other more favourable features. Hips showing two or more of these signs were designated 'at risk'. This category is now regarded by us as the most important for it over-rides the prognostic significance of individual groups.

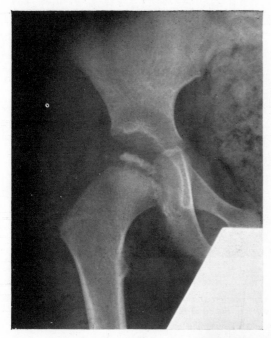

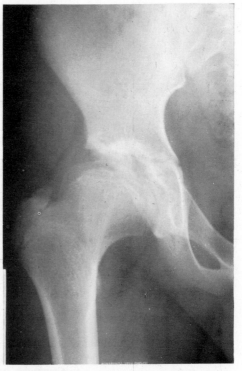

(a)

Figure 4.5. Group 4 Perthes' disease (Catterall classification). In spite of prolonged relief from weight-bearing the head is flattened and bulges laterally (Reproduced from Lloyd-Roberts, *Orthopaedics in Infancy and Childhood*, 1971)

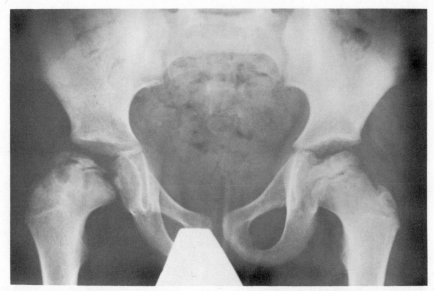

Figure 4.6. There is wide extrusion on the left and the acetabulum is beginning to adapt its contour to cover the displaced head. On the right the head remains contained within the acetabulum

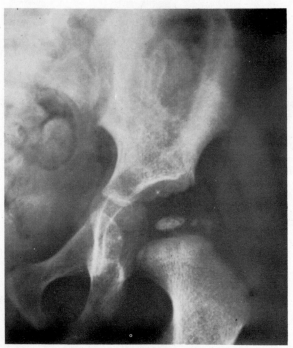

Figure 4.7. Calcification is seen lateral to the head which is itself somewhat extruded

130

Hips 'at risk' may display lateral subluxation (extrusion) (*Figure 4.6*) of the femoral head, speckled calcification lateral to the epiphysis (*Figure 4.7*), translucency at its lateral margin (*Figure 4.8*), diffuse metaphysial reaction and a horizontal growth plate. These signs may appear singly or in combination. Lateral extrusion is by far the most important for it warns of danger at an early stage, whereas the others are usually seen later when the head may already be deformed. Extrusion, alone, now prompts us to designate the hip 'at risk', whereas previously at least two signs were thought to be necessary.

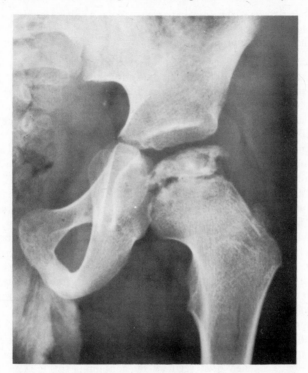

Figure 4.8. A translucent area is visible in the lateral part of the head (Gage's sign)

We believe that we now have a method of classification of sufficient reliability for us to compare the effects of different forms of treatment carried out in different centres, and this view is confirmed by Kamhi and MacEwen (1975). Assessment of results still requires standardization. Although we have preferred the simple good, fair and poor categorization, it may be preferable to use Mose's transparent template estimating the sphericity of the head in relation to circles drawn at expanding intervals or Eyre-Brooke's epiphyseal index. It is certainly unhelpful to compare the head shape at diagnosis with that at the stage of healing for the variables of group, duration of disease, and deformity in translucent cartilage, are more important than the apparent shape of the ossific nucleus as seen in the first radiograph. Furthermore some 50 per cent of unselected patients will have a satisfactory outcome without treatment.

In considering the choice of methods of treatment, we must be greatly influenced by this last factor and by earlier work which convinced us that protection from weight-bearing alone does nothing to protect the hip from deformation when it displays the features that would suggest that deformity is the likely outcome. In the next section, therefore, such methods will be discarded and the containment principle discussed in relation to the prognostic criteria which Catterall has established.

TREATMENT BY FEMORAL HEAD CONTAINMENT

The containment concept

Developments in our understanding of disease processes commonly progress on a wide front and Perthes' disease is not exceptional in this respect. Coincidentally with increasing knowledge of the natural history, radiological grouping, morbid anatomy etc., there arose a general disenchantment with the methods of treatment (or lack of it) in general use. We suspected that most of our efforts did little to influence the natural history of the disease and that some of the modes of treatment were, if not harmful, unjustifiable on social, financial and psychological grounds.

We also realized that the major impact of ischaemia was directed against the anterolateral segment of the femoral head and that this area was vulnerable to compression by the acetabular margin especially when there was some lateral extrusion. Clearly this segment weakened by ischaemia was likely to collapse under this abnormal pressure. Collapse leads to loss of epiphyseal height at the point naturally adapted to the greatest physiological loading. This alters the relative pressure on other normally non-pressure areas of the head which also tend to flatten if affected by ischaemia. Furthermore, the anterolateral zone is squeezed laterally so that when the area is revascularized and re-ossified part of the epiphysis will lie on the superior margin of the femoral neck. Thus we see the development of the mushroom head or, in extreme circumstances, a fracture of the epiphysis at the point of contact with the acetabular lip (*Figure 4.9*).

It was inevitable that consideration should be given to the possibility of protecting the weakened head segment by containing this area entirely within the cup of the acetabulum. If the leg is abducted and internally rotated the anterolateral segment is so protected and containment within the mould of the acetabulum achieved. McKibbin and Ralis (1974) have, on the basis of their postmortem observations, cast some doubt on this assumption because in their specimen the point of greatest depression of the head was central to the lateral edge of the epiphysis and apparently well within the acetabular cup. There was, however, some lateral extrusion in the non-weight-bearing radiograph, which would to some extent account for this. Of greater importance was the use of weight-relieving caliper for two years. Calipers cause further lateral extrusion which was well known in the days of poliomyelitis and has been confirmed by cineradiography in Perthes' disease. This implies that, on walking, the head was further extruded and if so the area of greatest compression might well have lain in contact with the lip of the acetabulum. There remains the possibility, however, that depression is due to contraction of fibrous tissue replacing necrotic trabeculae within the femoral head.

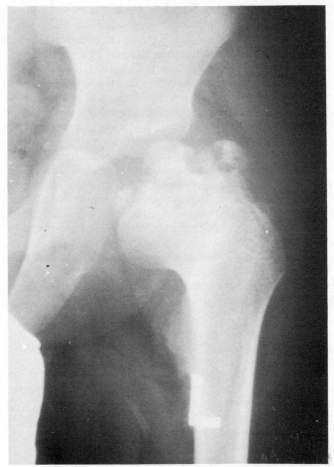

Figure 4.9. Severe Perthes' disease in which a fragment has become detached from the lateral side of the head due probably to compression by the acetabular rim

Although the containment concept is of great contemporary interest we should not forget that the principle was practised but not published by a few before the Second World War. Bristow certainly treated Perthes' disease in wide abduction on a frame and Parker used long leg plasters abducted by a cross-bar, to name but two of, perhaps, many.

Methods of containment

Two early methods have already been mentioned of which Parker's is still employed but the move away from prolonged in-patient treatment and the risk of immobilization porosis and subsequent capital collapse have relegated Bristow's method to history.

During recent years, several methods have been introduced to provide containment without the need for a long period of immobilization. These may be broadly divided into non-surgical and surgical. Examples of the former include plasters applied in abduction and internal rotation attached by broomsticks in which the child can walk with crutches (Petrie and Bitenc, 1971). Harrison's caliper splint is non-weight bearing and again maintains the leg in abduction and internal rotation (Harrison, Turner and Nicolson, 1969). Surgical methods obtain containment by either covering the head from above by innominate osteotomy (Salter, 1966; Canale *et al.*, 1972) or from below by means of a femoral varus rotation osteotomy which places the head deeply within the existing acetabulum (Axer, 1965, 1973; Somerville, 1971). All these reports share in common enthusiasm for the benefits of containment and indeed the published results are sufficiently encouraging, even without control series, to persuade us to accept that the principle has some virtue. Enthusiasm however should be tempered by the knowledge that 59 per cent of untreated patients will develop a good head shape (Catterall, 1971). Thus, in considering overall results of any form of treatment, we should regard a failure rate of more than 50 per cent as indicating that the method under review is not influencing significantly the natural history of the disease. Our criticism must therefore be directed towards the 40 per cent likely to do badly and our analysis towards a consideration of the effect of containment (or any other technique) upon these. This will be the approach used when describing controlled results following surgical containment.

The selection of method

If the surgeon decides to adopt the principle he must choose between the available methods. The first option is between splinting and surgery and, if surgery is chosen, between innominate and femoral osteotomy.

If splinting is selected and we assume (sometimes without total conviction) that the desired position can be both obtained and maintained, we must still submit the child to a much longer period of treatment than that required by surgical methods which average about 8 weeks in comparison with 84 weeks (Harrison) and 76 weeks (Petrie). Furthermore, the time at which the splint is removed and the femoral head submitted once more to acetabular pressure must involve a decision somewhat unsoundly based, for we do not know for certain at which stage the head is no longer vulnerable to deformation. By operating, however, we can arrange the relationship between head and acetabulum to our liking and, having done so, ensure by internal fixation that this is maintained indefinitely so that this difficult decision need no longer concern us. The case for operation is a strong one in an age when conservatism no longer merits the prestige it enjoyed in former days. We do not hesitate to perform similar operations in congenital dislocation when we wish to maintain congruity which is another word for containment. Why hesitate in Perthes' disease? Some favour a compromise, using a splint in young children who in general will have a better prognosis and reserving operation for the older. The validity of this will be discussed later.

If surgical treatment is selected we must now choose between the innominate and femoral osteotomy. We decided some years ago to adopt the femoral operation for a number of reasons. Firstly, it was possible to reproduce exactly both the degree of containment that could be achieved and the required angles of osteotomy by making a pre-operative radiograph in abduction and internal rotation (*Figure 4.10*). We could thus identify those in whom containment was no longer possible, and, having sometimes confirmed this by radiological examination (including arthrography) under anaesthesia with adductor tenotomy, withhold operation in unfavourable cases. We believed that less precision was possible prior to innominate osteotomy. Secondly, we were anxious lest innominate osteotomy should by its very nature impose some undesirable compression upon the femoral head — psoas tenotomy notwithstanding. The varus element of the femoral osteotomy and the slight shortening so produced can, on the other hand, be seen to decompress on the evidence of an increase in joint space in the postoperative radiograph. Thirdly, we find the femoral operation easier to perform and stabilize. It is also easier to correct later any technical error which may have been committed. Lastly, a study of the radiographs of patients submitted to innominate osteotomy appeared to show that sometimes the degree of coverage was less than one would have wished because of the technical limitations of the operation in this context. We still believe on the basis of further practical experience that these theoretical reasons for preferring the femoral operation remain valid — this is not to imply that excellent results cannot be achieved by innominate osteotomy but we lack comparative studies.

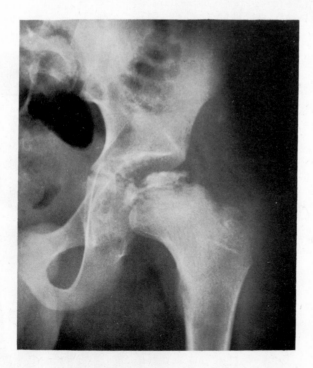

Figure 4.10. (a) There is extrusion and Gage's sign is present

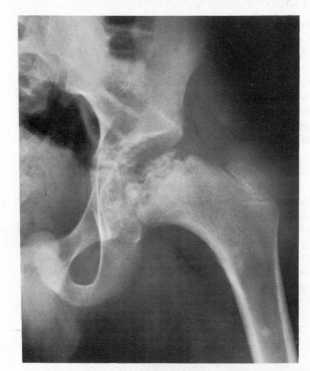

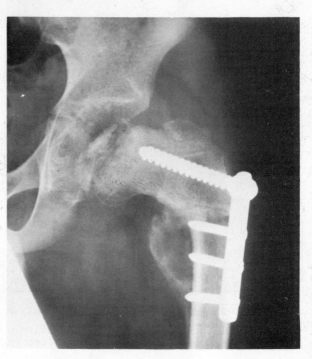

The management of those selected for containment using femoral osteotomy

Our present views upon the selection of patients will be presented later. These are based on our indiscriminate application of the method which exposed our errors initially.

Somerville (1971) has emphasized the importance of preliminary traction and plaster to improve the range of hip movement before operation. We have not followed this practice providing that adequate containment is possible when the leg is placed in that position of abduction and internal rotation that irritability of the hip permits. If uncertain, we have repeated the radiograph under anaesthesia before proceeding and have frequently noted an increase in joint movement sufficient to resolve the problem though adductor tenotomy may be necessary. The rest, enforced by the postoperative plaster, ensures that this improvement is maintained when the plaster is removed.

The method of fixation has varied for we have used angled plates, small fixed-angle nail plates and the Coventry lag screw and plate which is now our preference for routine use. A detailed description of the technique follows (*Figure 4.11*).

Following preliminary infiltration with 1/400 000 adrenaline with hyalase, the incision is made from just behind the anterior superior iliac spine curving across the tip of the trochanter to continue downwards in the line of the femur. The interval between gluteus medius and the tensor fascia is developed. Vastus lateralis is incised longitudinally, the incision above being carried medially to detach the part originating from the front of the trochanteric area. The calcar femorale may now be seen and the femoral head within the capsule can be felt. The hip is inwardly rotated as far as it will go and the guide wire inserted parallel to the floor in the lateral plate and to the calcar in the proximally-inclined oblique plane. The depth of penetration of the wire is of little importance but the selected lag screw should not encroach upon the palpable lateral margin of the head. The lag screw is inserted using the box spanner following drilling of the lateral cortex with a trephine. An oscillating saw is used to cut the femur at the intertrochanteric level parallel to the calcar using the guide wire which protrudes from the lag screw as the direction finder. The periosteum is stripped to allow free rotation of the distal fragment.

The guide wire is removed and the top hole of a straight plate is engaged to the protruding end of the lag screw which is grooved to accept the nut which finally secures the apposition of both. A suitably cannulated lever is screwed in place lateral to the plate with which the proximal fragment may be manipulated. By this means, we achieve abduction and medial rotation when the lever is parallel to the floor and the oblique osteotomy is realigned horizontally. The distal fragment is now laterally rotated until the patella points to the ceiling when the previously medial surface becomes anterior bringing forward a triangle of bone which the oblique osteotomy will inevitably create. This is excised if necessary and the fragments opposed and secured by screws below and by a nut above at the junction of plate and lag screw. The nut is tightened by the box spanner opposed by a conventional 'c' spanner which prevents rotation of the lag screw and the proximal fragment. Apposition and fixation will be found easier if performed with both fragments in some mutual flexion.

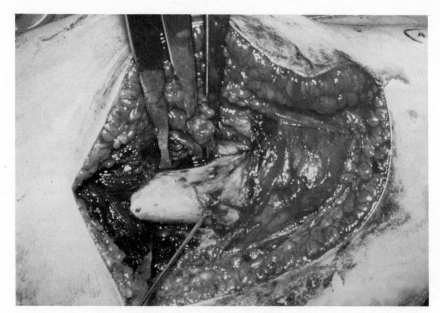

Figure 4.11. (a) The guide wire is inserted parallel to the floor and in the plane of the calcar femorale with the hip fully internally rotated

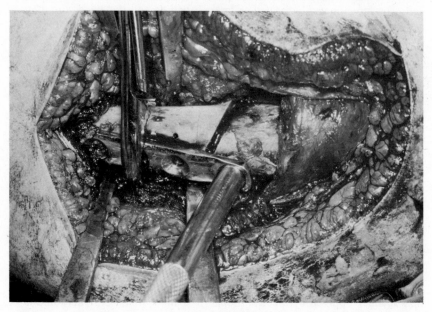

Figure 4.11. (b) The osteotomy has been made and the proximal fragment is held in abduction and internal rotation. The distal fragment is externally rotated, opposed to the proximal and secured in this position

Fixation is secure but plaster is used, because the child may then usually be discharged home within two to three days which is economically of benefit and, in accordance with contemporary teaching, beneficial to the psyche. Without plaster, pain on movement and anxiety will delay discharge for some ten days.

The child is re-admitted six weeks later for removal of the plaster and to check the soundness of union and the degree of containment. Within two to three days we expect the knee and hip to flex to right angles and then walking is allowed. We somewhat piously suggest that rough games, jumping from a height, etc. be avoided for six months but, in most, these regulations are uninforceable.

In ideal circumstances we would remove the metal in six months but pressure on beds precludes this unless the nut is prominent and painful beneath the skin. This is the only disadvantage of the method and it is a common problem even when care is taken during closure to cover the nut with as thick a layer of muscle as possible. The other 'disadvantage' is excess shortening due to the varus component of the osteotomy — a complication not arising after innominate osteotomy. This used to concern us but we now know that it is seldom severe and usually temporary for 26 patients studied specifically in this context had on average 2 cm of shortening less than 6 years after operation but only 1.25 cm over 6 years — a discrepancy compatible with that attributable to the disease itself. It has not been necessary to repeat the operation because of loss of congruity with further growth and only 1 patient has required re-admission and traction for unexplained postoperative irritability.

The controlled results of containment by femoral osteotomy

We, (Lloyd-Roberts, Catterall and Salamon, 1976) have recently reported these results in detail and I will therefore only describe them in general terms and give a summary of our present attitudes.

Having accepted the principle in 1963, we applied it by femoral osteotomy to all patients except those in whom it was impossible to achieve containment in the pre-operative radiograph. In our review, however, we excluded some for the following reasons. Firstly, half-head disease (O'Garra, 1959; Catterall, 1971, Group 1) evidently required no treatment; secondly, uncertainty about the relative importance of the biological (vascular) and the mechanical nature of the effects of operation led us in some to omit internal fixation; thirdly, the earliest operations did not include the medial rotation component so that the zone of the greatest impact of the disease remained unprotected; and lastly, in a few we had been overenthusiastic in operating upon patients in whom the changes were so advanced that no form of treatment was likely to influence the outcome.

There remained 48 hips categorized as Catterall Group 2, 3 or 4 in whom full containment was possible in the pre-operative radiograph, followed for at least 4 years after operation with an average of 6 years.

The controls

The importance of controls has already been emphasized and for this purpose we used two series: first, untreated patients (75 hips), and second, patients treated by either a caliper alone or following a period of bed-rest of not more than four months (95 hips). It is evident that neither series involved containment. Both excluded Group 1 but of course failure to contain in an early radiograph did not apply.

There was no difference in outcome between these control series both showing overall results radiologically inferior to those of containment.

TABLE 4.III

To show that there is no difference in outcome between untreated patients and those treated by methods not involving containment. The results of osteotomy are superior to both. (Reproduced from Lloyd-Roberts, Catterall and Salamon (1976) by permission)

	Good		Fair		Poor	
	Number	%	Number	%	Number	%
Osteotomies	28	58	11	23	9	19
Untreated controls	32	43	21	28	22	29
Uncontained treated controls	44	46	25	26	26	28

It is clear that this method not involving containment had no influence on the natural history of the disease. The difference between 43 per cent spontaneous good results and the 59 per cent previously quoted is explained by the exclusion of Group 1 disease. This similarity enabled us to use untreated patients only as our controls.

The results

We classified our results on radiological criteria as good, fair and poor. Good hips remained fully contained having a spherical epiphysis of normal or good height (*Figure 4.12*). The fair were congruous, up to 1/5 of an inch uncovered with more loss of epiphyseal height (*Figure 4.13*). Poor were worse than this and included hips with flattening, lack of cover, extrusion and secondary acetabular adaptation (*Figure 4.14*).

(a) *Overall results in Group 2, 3, 4*   These are shown in Table 4.III and display a margin in favour of containment.

(b) *Results related to group*   These disclosed that containment conferred no benefit in Group 2 but seemed to do so modestly in Groups 3 and 4 (Table 4.IV).

(c) *Results related to age*   There was a balance in favour of containment when applied over the age of 6 years but this was also evident in younger children to a lesser degree (Table 4.V).

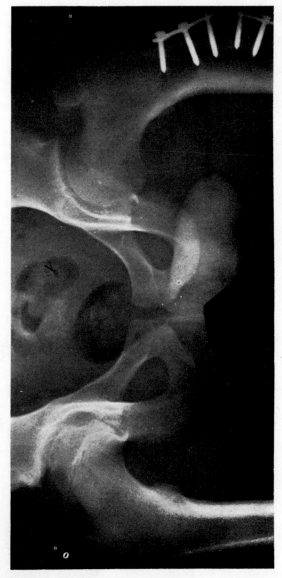

Figure 4.12. A good result. The head retains its height, is fully contained and spherical following subtrochanteric osteotomy with plate fixation. (Reproduced from Lloyd-Roberts, Catterall and Salaman (1976) by permission)

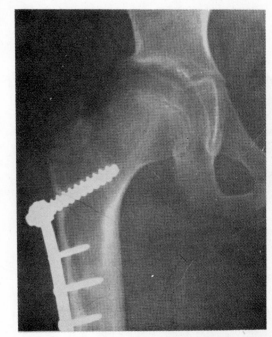

Figure 4.13. A fair result. There is some loss of head height with some loss of containment but the contour is spherical. Intertrochanteric osteotomy with Coventry fixation device (Reproduced from Lloyd-Roberts, Catterall and Salaman (1976) by permission)

Figure 4.14. A poor result. The head is flattened, deformed and poorly covered. The neck is short and wide. (Reproduced from Lloyd-Roberts, Catterall and Salaman (1976) by permission)

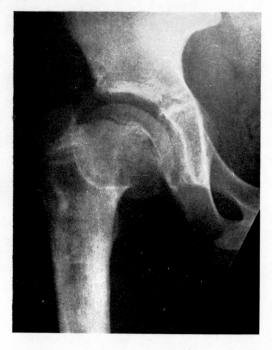

TABLE 4.IV

The results of containment osteotomy compared with those in untreated patients related to disease groups. (Reproduced by permission from Lloyd-Roberts, Catterall and Salaman (1976))

The results of osteotomy related to group

Group	Patients	Good Number	%	Fair Number	%	Poor Number	%
2	19	16	84	2	11	1	5
3	20	7	35	8	40	5	25
4	9	5	56	1	11	3	33

The results of no treatment related to group

Group	Patients	Good Number	%	Fair Number	%	Poor Number	%
2	33	26	79	5	15	2	6
3	25	5	20	9	36	11	44
4	17	1	6	7	41	9	53

TABLE 4.V

The results of osteotomy related to age of operation. (Reproduced by permission from Lloyd-Roberts, Catterall and Salaman (1976))

Results of osteotomy performed over the age of six years compared with untreated controls

	Patients	Good Number	%	Fair Number	%	Poor Number	%
Osteotomies	24	12	50	5	21	7	29
Controls	25	7	28	9	36	9	36

Results of osteotomy performed under the age of six years compared with untreated controls

	Patients	Good Number	%	Fair Number	%	Poor Number	%
Osteotomies	24	16	66	6	25	2	9
Controls	50	25	50	12	24	13	26

(d) *Results related to 'at risk' signs*   The signs upon which the assessment of 'at risk' is made have already been described and in view of their influence upon outcome to be reported below we now regard these factors to be of paramount importance.

Table 4.VI shows that 'at risk factors' in untreated patients dominate the outcome in Groups 3 and 4 and influence it considerably in Group 2. Overall, 71 per cent of those hips not 'at risk' developed a good shape whereas, if 'at risk', this fell to 31 per cent – when operation was performed on those 'at risk', 53 per cent had a good result, whereas operation did not influence the outcome in hips 'at risk' for the incidence of good results remains at 71 per cent.

Summarizing the effects of containment upon the natural history we find that the method greatly improves the outcome in those 'at risk' but it has little or no influence on those with no such stigmata. Furthermore, this influence dominates prognosis not only between the groups but also concerning the factor of age.

Miscellaneous observations on results

(1) *The outcome in all groups*   In considering the outcome in all groups we must remember that if any form of treatment fails to produce a satisfactory outcome in more than 50 per cent of cases overall we should regard the method as having an insignificant influence upon the natural history of the disease. In Table 4.III containment is shown to be followed by good results in only 58 per cent and no treatment by good results in 43 per cent, but this excludes patients with Group 1 disease which invariably has a good prognosis. The incidence of Group 1 disease is about 30 per cent of all patients (Catterall, 1971). If we add this proportion to our figures for Group 2, 3 and 4 as shown in Table 4.VII, we can estimate the influence of containment expressed as overall results for all groups.

If we compare the good results we find a 20 per cent advantage in favour of containment over the expected 50 per cent. Of more significance, perhaps, is the fact that the poor results are halved.

(2) *Predicting final results*   In predicting final results it must be emphasized that the average age of our patients at review was 12 years and the follow-up period 6 years, so that most have not reached maturity and clearly our results are intermediate. However, Somerville (1971) has shown that well contained heads continue to improve with time and we have confirmed this observation in a separate study of 64 hips reviewed more than 10 years after primary healing. It is likely, therefore, that some of the hips categorized as 'fair' will be promoted to 'good' with time, producing a further improvement in overall results. This is probable when the joint space remains wide at the end of primary healing.

(3) *Withholding operation in the very young*   Some surgeons withhold operation in patients with early-onset disease preferring not to treat them or to use abduction splinting. Comparison between the results before and after 6 years does not

TABLE 4.VI

To show the significance of 'at risk' factors in relation to the outcome in treated and untreated patients. (Reproduced from Lloyd-Roberts, Catterall and Salaman (1976) by permission)

The results of osteotomy related to 'at risk' factors present

Group	Patients	Good Number	Good %	Fair Number	Fair %	Poor Number	Poor %
2	10	9	90	–	–	1	10
3	17	6	35	7	41	4	24
4	7	3	43	1	14	3	43
Totals	34	18	53	8	23.5	8	23.5

The results of osteotomy related to 'at risk' factors absent

Group	Patients	Good Number	Good %	Fair Number	Fair %	Poor Number	Poor %
2	9	7	77	2	23	–	–
3	3	1	33	1	33	1	33
4	2	2	100	–	–	–	–
Totals	14	10	71	3	21	1	7

The results with no treatment related to 'at risk' factors present

Group	Patients	Good Number	Good %	Fair Number	Fair %	Poor Number	Poor %
2	19	14	73	3	16	2	11
3	20	3	15	6	30	11	55
4	15	–	–	6	40	9	60
Totals	54	17	31	15	28	22	41

The results of no treatment related to 'at risk' factors absent

Group	Patients	Good Number	Good %	Fair Number	Fair %	Poor Number	Poor %
2	14	12	86	2	14	–	–
3	5	2	40	3	60	–	–
4	2	1	50	1	50	–	–
Totals	21	15	71	6	29	–	–

TABLE 4.VII
Projected results including Group I

	Number	% good	% fair	% poor
Osteotomies	62	70	18	12
No treatment	97	50	25	25

support this proposition for youth does not protect a hip with 'at risk' signs though of course the incidence of hips at risk is less in the younger children.

(4) *The rate of re-ossification*   Following operation we sometimes see a rapid and remarkable change in the femoral head which suggests that healing is accelerating (Axer, 1965). Recently, in a careful study using controls, Marklund and Tillberg (1976) have shown that this is in general an illusion but they support Harrison's observation that when osteotomy is performed late in the evolution of the disease there is a slightly higher rate of re-ossification.

(5) *The timing of operation*   This is clearly of great importance when the outcome is destined to be poor, for all such hips must at some stage reach a point of no return when deformity prevents congruous containment. Studies of arthrograms made some years ago showed that there was an appreciable time lag between collapse of the ossific nucleus and that of the overlying epiphyseal cartilage.

This is fortunate in many ways for we are unable in the early stages to categorize a hip into one or other group and to decide whether or not to classify the hip as being 'at risk'. Furthermore, we are frequently unsure of the duration of the disease when the patient is first seen because of the variability in the relationship between the time of onset of the disease and the onset of symptoms – this is particularly true in the younger children.

Our results suggest, as an approximation, that 7 months from the onset of symptoms is the critical time, for our good results averaged 7½ and fair 6½ months between onset and operation. We are therefore entitled to a waiting period of observation in many patients but whether we should protect these hips in an abduction splint or simply monitor by periodic radiographs remains unresolved. Hitherto we have not treated them.

Poor results averaged 21 months from the onset of symptoms and, on critical retrospective review, we concluded that we had sometimes operated unwisely when irreversible deformity was probably already present. Overlooked secondary acetabular adaptation was often the cause of our error.

Operating at this late stage is certainly useless and may well be harmful. The relatively good long-term prognosis even in the presence of head flattening may well be due to the acetabulum adapting itself, during further growth, to the shape of the head so that a state of 'incongruous congruity' is reached. To alter this relationship between head and acetabulum once structural adaptation has begun may be to produce a situation of 'incongruous incongruity' which is unlikely to be of benefit to the patient (Curtis, 1972). This may be expressed alternatively as 'regular or irregular congruity', i.e. provided an irregular head is matched by an irregular acetabulum the prognosis may be unexpectedly good.

A margin of success no greater than 20 per cent over the expected incidence is not sensational. Nevertheless, our proportion of good results will rise as we learn how to exclude unfavourable hips and as, we hope, some existing results are promoted in grade.

Lastly, if operation does no more than reduce treatment time from 1 to 2 years to 8 weeks without detriment it will be fully justified.

Conclusions

Conscious of perhaps having overstated out own views which are based on a relatively small number of patients, our recommendations must be advanced with caution for we have still much to learn. For example, we know little of the long-term outlook for these patients though we may hope that this will depend upon the quality of the head contour and hip congruity at the end of primary healing (Helbo, 1953). Our suggestions for selecting patients for containment require confirmation or rebuttal and observations upon the timing of operation are but speculative.

The criteria proposed to identify those hips 'at risk' are in general valid but we must concede a significant margin of error. Thus, of those so described but untreated, 30 per cent developed satisfactorily, the outcome being classified as good (Table 4.VI). If we are to accept the 'at risk' factor as paramount we must critically re-examine these criteria seeking for the clues which will enable us to make the diagnosis with greater precision.

We have still to assess the influence of relief from weight-bearing in relation to containment. Our patients were not so protected once containment was achieved, but it is important that a comparable study be mounted combining containment with weight-relief. McKibbin tells me that this is at present under investigation. The patients under review are those treated by Parker many years ago in whom prolonged bed-rest was combined with abduction plasters. The preliminary results suggest that this combination achieves better results than those of containment alone in Group 4 disease.

Lastly, little has been said about the cause and effect of premature arrest of the capital growth plate. This is a serious complication and we must try to relate it to both types of disease and the methods of treatment employed.

The important development in recent years is the progress towards an increasing awareness of the need to obtain an agreed classification of the disease and agreed criteria of late assessment. Once these are accepted we can advance for we will thus be able to compare the results obtained by different methods in several centres. Within these limitations, however, our tentative conclusions and recommendations at the present time are as follows.

(1) The principle of containment is sound and should be offered in some form to some patients.

(2) It is probable that modes of treatment which do not involve containment do not influence the natural history of the disease.

(3) There is no evidence that containment is of benefit to those for whom it is not indicated.

REFERENCES

(4) Containment by femoral varus and internal rotation osteotomy is a satisfactory technique of achieving and maintaining containment and preferable to non-operative methods.

(5) Containment by femoral osteotomy is indicated at all ages when there is radiological evidence of the epiphysis being 'at risk' to deformation and this should be employed within 7 months of the onset of symptoms.

(6) Treatment should be withheld when:
   (a) the epiphysis is graded as Group 1;
   (b) the epiphysis is not 'at risk';
   (c) deformation of the epiphysis or acetabulum prevents congruous containment.

REFERENCES

Axer, A. (1965). Subtrochanteric osteotomy in the treatment of Perthes' Disease. *J. Bone Jt Surg.* **47B,** 489

Axer, A., Sculler, M. G., Segal, D., Rzetelny, V., and Gershuni-Gordon, D. H. (1973). Subtrochanteric osteotomy in the treatment of Legg–Calvé–Perthes syndrome. *Acta Orth. Scand.* **44,** 31

Brown, I. (1975). A study of the 'capsular' shadow in disorders of the hip in children. *J. Bone Jt Surg.* **57B,** 175

Canale, S. T., D'Anca, A. F., Cotler, J. M., and Snedden, H. E. (1972). Innominate osteotomy in Legg–Calvé–Perthes Disease. *J. Bone Jt Surg.* **54A,** 25

Catterall, A. (1971). The natural history of Perthes' Disease. *J. Bone Jt Surg.* **53B,** 37

Catterall, A., Lloyd-Roberts, G. C. and Wynne-Davies, Ruth. (1971). Association of Perthes' Disease with congenital anomalies of genito-urinary tract and inguinal region. *Lancet,* May 15,

Curtis, (1972). Personal communication

Evans, D. L. and Lloyd-Roberts, G. C. (1958). Treatment in Legg–Calvé–Perthes Disease. A comparison of in-patient and out-patient methods. *J. Bone Jt Surg.* **40B,** 182

Ferguson, A. B. and Howarth, M. B. (1934). Coxa plana and related conditions at the hip. *J. Bone Jt Surg.* **16,** 781

Fisher, R. L. (1972). An epidemiological study of Legg–Perthes Disease. *J. Bone Jt Surg.* **54A,** 769

Goff, C. W. (1954). *Legg–Calvé–Perthes Syndrome and Related Osteochondrosis of Young Children.* Springfield, Illinois: Charles C. Thomas

Harrison, M. H. M., Turner, M. H. and Jacobs, P. (1976). Skeletal immaturity in Perthes' Disease. *J. Bone Jt Surg.* **58B,** 37

Harrison, M. H. M., Turner, M. H. and Nicholson, F. J. (1969). Coxa plana – results of a new form of splinting. *J. Bone Jt Surg.* **51A,** 1057

Helbo, S. (1953). *Morbo Calvé Perthe.* Odense: Fyns Tidendes

Hipp, E. (1962). Perthes' Disease. *Z. Orthop.* **Suppl. 96**

Kamhi, E. and MacEwen, G. D. (1975). Osteochondritis dissecans in Legg–Calvé–Perthes Disease. *J. Bone Jt. Surg.* **57A,** 506

Kamhi, E. and MacEwen, G. D. (1975). Treatment of Legg-Calvé–Perthes Disease. *J. Bone Jt Surg.* **57A,** 651

Kemp, H. B. S. (1973). Perthes' Disease. An experimental and clinical study. *Ann. R. Coll. Surg.* **52,** 18

Kemp, H. B. S. and Baijens, J. K. (1971). Recurrent Perthes' Disease. *Br. J. Radiol.* **44,** 675

Lloyd-Roberts, G. C., Catterall, A., and Salaman, P. B. (1976). A controlled study of the indications for and the results of femoral osteotomy in Perthes' Disease. *J. Bone Jt Surg.* **58B,** 31

Marklund, T. and Tillberg, B. (1976). Coxa Plana. A radiological comparison of the rate of healing with conservative measures and after osteotomy. *J. Bone Jt. Surg.* **58B,** 25

McKibbin, B. (1975). Recent developments in Perthes' Disease in *Recent Advances in Orthopaedics.* p. 173. London: Churchill Livingstone

REFERENCES

McKibbin, B. and Ralis, Z. (1974). Pathological changes in a case of Perthes' Disease. *J. Bone Jt Surg.* **56B,** 438

Morley, T. (1975). Unpublished work

Murley, A. H. G. and Lloyd-Roberts, G. C. (1962). Unpublished work

O'Garra, J. A. (1959). The radiographic changes in Perthes' Disease. *J. Bone Jt Surg.* **41B,** 465

Petrie, J. G. and Bitenc, I. (1971). The abduction weight-bearing treatment in Legg–Perthes Disease. *J. Bone Jt Surg.* **53B,** 54

Ponsetti, I. V. (1956). Legg–Perthes Disease. Observations on pathological changes in two cases. *J. Bone Jt Surg.* **38A,** 739

Ratliff, A. H. C. (1967a). Perthes' Disease. A study of 34 hips observed for 30 years. *J. Bone Jt Surg.* **49B,** 102

Ratliff, A. H. C. (1967b). Osteochondritis dissecans following Legg–Calvé–Perthes Disease. *J. Bone Jt Surg.* **49B,** 108

Robichon, J., Desjardins, J. P., Koch, M., and Hooper, C. E. (1974). The femoral neck in Legg–Perthes Disease. Its relationship to epiphyseal change and its importance in early prognosis. *J. Bone Jt Surg.* **54A,** 62

Salter, R. B. (1966). Experimental and clinical aspects of Perthes' Disease. *J. Bone Jt Surg.* **48B,** 393

Salter, R. B. (1966). Legg–Perthes Disease. *J. Bone Jt Surg.* **48B,** 854

Sanchis, M., Zahir, A., and Freeman, M. A. R. (1973). The experimental simulation of Perthes' Disease by consecutive interruptions of the blood supply to the capital femoral epiphysis in the puppy. *J. Bone Jt Surg.* **55A,** 335

Somerville, E. W. (1971). Perthes' Disease of the hip. *J. Bone Jt Surg.* **53B,** 639

Spivey, J. and Park, W. M. (1973). The production of ischaemic lesions in the hips of immature rabbits using arterial microemboli. *J. Bone Jt. Surg.* **55B,** 655

Suramo, I., Puranen, J., Heikkenen, E. and Vuorinen, P. (1974). Disturbed patterns of venous drainage of the femoral neck in Perthes' Disease. *J. Bone Jt Surg.* **56B,** 448

4

Perthes' Disease–Part II
The Long-Term Results

A. H. C. Ratliff

In this section discussion will be entirely concentrated on our present knowledge of long-term results of Perthes' disease in the adult. It is perhaps agreed that the ultimate criterion on which success of the various methods of treatment must be judged is the clinical and radiological condition in the adult observed for probably 40 years or more. Only then will sufficient time have elapsed for possible secondary osteoarthritis to develop and for the results of different methods of treatment to be compared. The discussion will be considered under four headings:

1. A review of previous studies;
2. A recent study of 16 hips observed for an average of 41 years (1976);
3. A study of cases classified as 'head at risk' and observed for 30 years;
4. Conclusions.

1. REVIEW OF THE LITERATURE

In the literature on such a perplexing subject it is surprising that there are relatively few reports of cases observed into adult life. Precise comparison of results in the adult is difficult, for many patients show full movements and normal activity, despite varying degrees of radiological abnormality. Most of the published series are bedevilled by one fact: they make no clear distinction between radiological osteoarthritis (i.e. a curious-shaped head with loss of joint space) and clinical osteoarthritis (i.e. pain and stiffness). Danielsson and Hernborg (1965); Ratliff (1956 and 1967); Eaton (1967) and Gower and Johnston (1971) all came to similar conclusions. Danielsson and Hernborg examined clinically and radiologically patients 33 years after the onset. 'In twenty-eight patients the hips were painless. Structural changes and/or narrowing of the joint space were noted in seventeen cases'. In Ratliff's series of 34 cases, 25 of whom had been treated by prolonged immobilization on frames and observed for an average of 30 years, 4 out of 5 patients were fully active and free from pain but only 2 out of 5 had hips which were radiologically good. In Eaton's series of 100 hips observed for an average of 19 years and treated in bed with or without traction, 64 per cent were classified as good but the assessment appeared to be largely clinical. Gower and Johnston (1971) noted that only 3 out of the 36 patients in their series had sufficient pain and impairment of function to require surgery in later life. The radiological results are described but the combined assessment of both clinical and radiological is not given. It would also appear from these studies that significant deterioration in function or radiological appearance was rare, at least up to 40 years of age.

The most important factor in prognosis appeared to be the age at onset. All children less than 5 years old and treated on a frame, and presumably therefore in some abduction, obtained good results. Apart from this is was not possible to predict accurately late results of Perthes' disease in adult life. The nature and growth of the head and neck of the femur with remodelling could not be forecast and occasionally produced unexpected results. This author was often surprised to note in his study the good clinical condition that had been maintained by so many patients. These long-term reviews, however, provide limited information since there are insufficient numbers of cases treated in precisely the same way and exact information on the method of adult assessment is not always given.

It must be emphasized that these papers were published before the important work of Catterall (1971 and 1972) whose classification of four degrees of severity of involvement of the upper femoral epiphysis is now well known. Nevertheless, the difficulty with the Catterall classification is that cases are not defined in terms of degree of involvement at the time of onset of the disease but rather one or two years later. The value of this classification is to some degree retrospective rather than prospective (Salter, et al., 1976). More recently, Brotherton and McKibbin (1976) have reported a long-term review of 102 hips observed for an average of 17 years. All the patients had been treated in wide abduction until fragmentation ceased and then in broomstick plasters with the hips abducted and internally rotated. They were supervised in hospital and the average time of splint immobilization was 26 months. Weight-bearing was not permitted. The results of treatment were better than those described by Ratliff (1956) who had assessed the results depending on the combination of four parameters, namely pain, activity, movement and radiological appearances. In Brotherton's paper 88 per cent were good, 10 per cent fair and only 2 per cent poor.

Salter (1976) considered that the most significant problem in Perthes' disease was the possibility of development of late arthritis. He and his colleagues from Toronto reported a long-term study of 34 adults with an average age of onset of 7 years and treated in a weight-relieving brace. The length of follow-up was 36 years and the average age at time of assessment was 43 years. Four observations were made. First, only those with significant radiological deformity, i.e. flattening of the femoral head, were likely to develop arthritis. Second, with residual significant deformity, the incidence of late arthritis varied directly with the age of onset of the Perthes' disease. If the onset was before the age of 6 years then arthritis never developed, if it commenced between 6 and 9 years the incidence was 40 per cent, and if the disease occurred over 10 years the incidence was 100 per cent. Third, in an investigation of the significance of the residual abnormality in the hip in relation to the arthritis, femoral-head deformity was significant whereas decreased epiphyseal height, coxa magna, and functional coxa vara were not significant. Finally, he considered that femoral-head deformity was usually preventable whereas decreased epiphyseal height, coxa magna and functional coxa vara were part of the natural course of severe Perthes' disease and were not preventable. He stressed that the age of onset, severity of disease, loss of containment and limitation of movement, especially abduction, were important. Features which were not significant were metaphyseal cysts, lateral calcification and the angle of the epiphyseal plate. However, it is noted that this paper contained no observations concerning the clinical conditions of the patients and his study was essentially radiological.

2. A STUDY OF 16 HIPS OBSERVED FOR AN AVERAGE OF 41 YEARS (1976)

This work is based on a further analysis of patients previously described (Ratliff 1956; 1967a, b). The shortest period of follow-up was 36 years and the longest 47 years. All patients seen at the time of the last review were circulated and every endeavour made to see them, but for various reasons this was not always possible and will not be further discussed. Most patients were seen by me, but in a few cases I am grateful to colleagues reporting the present state. Ten of the

TABLE 4.VIII
A review of 16 hips in 15 patients (11 men, 4 women) and followed for 41 years

Ages of patients	39–55 years	(average 47)
Length of follow-up	35–47 years	(average 41)
Good hips	(18–20 points)	5
Fair hips	(15–17 points)	6
Poor or very poor hips	(14 or less points)	5

Details (one excluded as surgery performed recently)

Pain	None or slight aches	13
Activity	Normal	9
Movement	Full or terminal restriction	7
Radiographs	Normal or slight flattening	5

hips had been treated by prolonged immobilization on frames, presumably in slight abduction, for an average period of 17 months. Six hips were untreated during the active phase of the disease, though sometimes receiving a period of immobilization in hospital when the femoral head was partly reformed; these are classified as untreated. The results of the 16 hips are shown in Table 4.VIII.

The assessment of results was carried out in the same way as previously (Brotherton and McKibbin, 1976; Ratliff, 1956 and 1967); it should be recalled that this classification is demanding as it expects a hip to obtain 18 points out of 20 to be classified as good and this is a considerable requirement for patients of

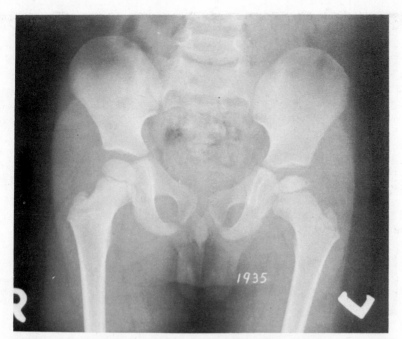

Figure 4.15. Illustrating an excellent result as expected; Grade 2, not 'at risk'.
(a) Radiograph when aged 4 in 1935. Treatment frame fixation 14 months

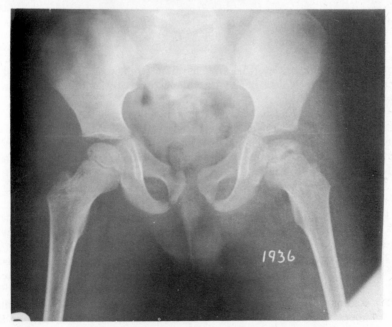

Figure 4.15. (b) Radiograph in 1936. Upper femoral epiphysis a little flattened
but well contained

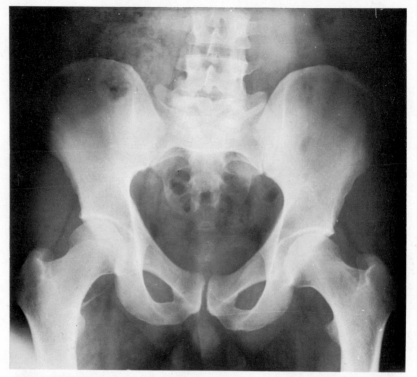

Figure 4.15. (c) Radiograph in 1976. A normal hip, no symptoms or signs. Was treatment necessary?

about 50 years of age. Nevertheless, it has been retained as the only method of comparison with previous studies. An example of an excellent result is shown in *Figure 4.15*.

It will be seen in this miscellaneous group of treated and untreated cases of Perthes' disease with a follow-up average of 41 years that approximately one-third were good, one-third were fair and one-third poor. As in the previous assessment relatively few patients suffered from pain or reduced activity but only one-third had good hips radiologically.

A comparison has been made with the condition in 1964 and in 1976:

1.   One patient previously classified as poor has had a total hip replacement performed. This is the only patient of these 16 in whom surgery has even been discussed.
2.   Slight symptomatic deterioration in the form of short episodes of pain, sometimes lasting for a few days, was mentioned by 3 patients but in none was it important and medical advice had not been sought.
3.   Radiological deterioration was noted in 5 patients, the outstanding impression being that these changes were slight and found only by the critical observer. Two of these patients mentioned symptomatic deterioration. None had attended hospital during the last 12 years except for the

1 total hip replacement. Thus it may be concluded that, with the rare exception of the occasional very poor result in late adolescence (Ratliff, 1956), a considerable proportion of cases of Perthes' disease observed up to about 50 years of age will have a satisfactory clinical result, even though there is significant radiological abnormality. With two exceptions — one who had an arthrodesis in 1954 and another who had an arthroplasty in 1973 — even those technically graded as poor did not require orthopaedic consultation or consider surgery.

The radiological appearance of Perthes' disease in adult life

Salter *et al.* (1976) have stressed that the most significant problem in Perthes' disease is the onset of late arthritis but the author has found the exact definition of this term difficult. Poor anatomical results were present in two-thirds of these 16 hips, illustrated in *Figures 4.16(c, d), 4.17(c)* and *4.19(c)*. Nevertheless, there does seem to be a characteristic appearance of incongruous congruity in adult life, where joint space is maintained, though with a large femoral head and short femoral neck. Deterioration at least up to the age of 50 does not appear to occur in these cases. Catterall (1972) has stressed that a small amount of lateral subluxation allows considerable uncovering of the femoral head and this process of subluxation is not lateral but anterolateral. This probably explains the oval rather than the rounded cavity of the acetabulum and the characteristic increased anteversion of the femoral neck (*Figure 4.16, c, d*).

Though children are seldom immobilized for long periods in hospital at the present time the possible psychological effects of this method of treatment were noted in this study. These 15 adult patients were questioned and asked to comment on the effect of their treatment from this point of view. The conclusions were quite clear: one patient stated that for some years in adolescence he was terrified of the possibility of having to return to in-patient treatment; but otherwise none had complaints in this respect. They all appeared well adjusted, balanced personalities and had not suffered from problems of depression or consulted psychiatrists. It must be pointed out that they were treated in hospitals with a well organized educational school service. None appeared to recall their period in hospital with anything but affection and many were especially co-operative in travelling long distances for the consultation necessary for this study.

The unaffected hip in patients with unilateral Perthes' disease

In 3 patients followed-up for 41 years there was one unexpected observation. Osteoarthritis with deformity and osteophyte formation was noted to be developing in the hip where radiographs demonstrated no abnormality in childhood. One of these 3 patients mentioned the problem of this hip and there were symptoms in relation to it. In the other 2 patients there were no symptoms. It is not proposed to discuss this matter in detail but it raises the controversial

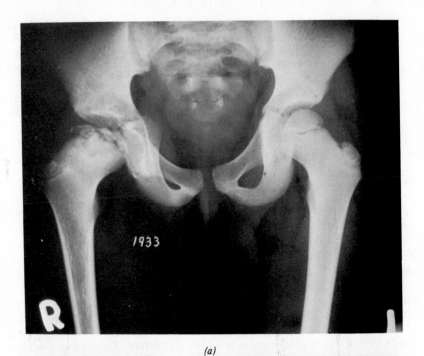

(a)

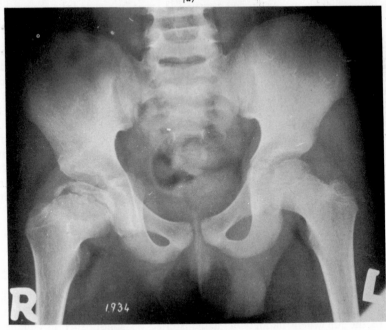

(b)

Figure 4.16. An example of an untreated case. (a) Radiograph of a boy aged 9 on admission in 1933. Catterall Group 3. Lateral calcification, head at risk. (b) Radiograph 8 months later, head not fully contained

156

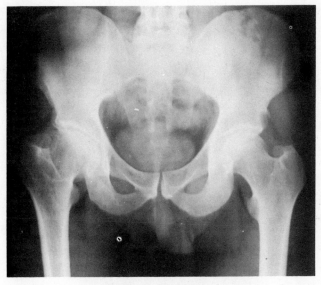

(c)

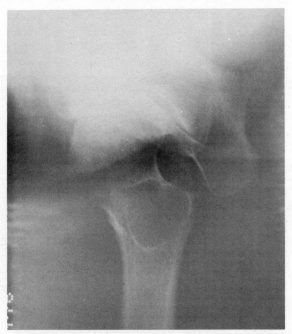

(d)

Figure 4.16. (c) and (d) Radiographs in 1976 when aged 52.
Minor aches, half-inch of shortening, some thigh wasting,
working capacity not affected as a foreman

157

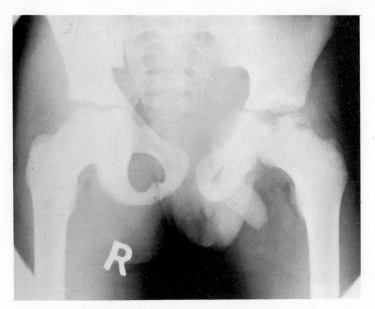

Figure 4.17. The development of arthritis in the unaffected hip. (a) A radiograph of a boy aged 7 on admission in 1930; only the left hip is involved; Catterall Group 3 – no treatment

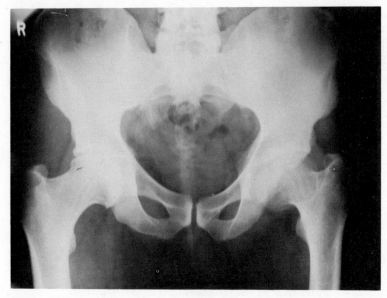

Figure 4.17. (b) Radiograph in February 1965. Note the apparently normal right hip

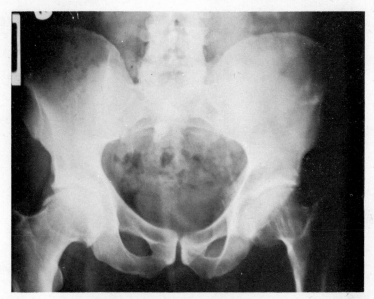

Figure 4.17. (c) Radiograph in 1976 when aged 53. Works as a grocer. No symptoms left hip. Osteoarthritis in right hip with some pain

subject of the unknown factors which cause possible malformation and presumably osteoarthritis of the hip joint in adults. Lloyd-Roberts (1955) noted that in 124 cases of osteoarthritis of the hip requiring surgery, 73 had an unknown cause and 3 followed Perthes' disease. An example is shown in *Figure 4.17.*

3. A STUDY OF 'HEAD AT RISK' OBSERVED FOR 30 YEARS

Of those cases observed for 30 years an analysis has been made of 14 classified as head at risk, out of a total of 28 observed where accurate documentation at the beginning of treatment was available. The results are shown in Table 4.IX (9 were treated and 5 untreated).

TABLE 4.IX
Results of cases classified as 'head at risk' observed for an average of 30 years

	Good	Fair	Poor
Treated (average 17 months)	3	4	2
Untreated	–	3	2

Limited conclusions only can be drawn from the analysis of a relatively small number, but it would appear that this study supports the concept that the radiological signs of a 'head at risk' are important in the prognosis of Perthes' disease. It will be noted that of 9 patients who had treatment 7 were free of

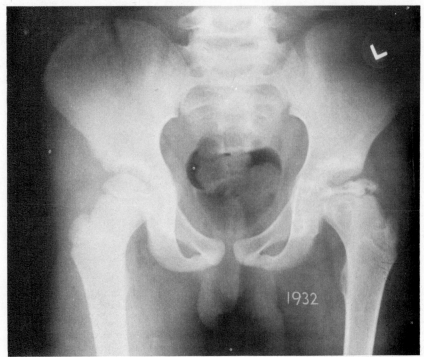

(4.18a)

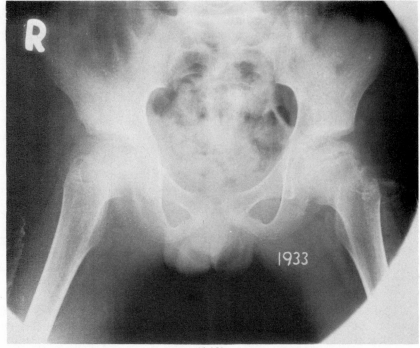

(4.18b)

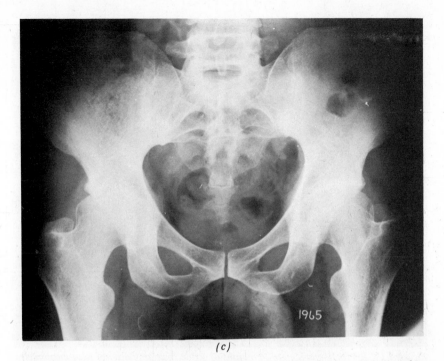

(c)

Figure 4.18. Illustrating an unexpected good result. (a) Radiograph on admission when 9 years old showing head at risk. (b) Radiograph after frame fixation for 14 months. Flattened epiphysis but well contained. (c) Radiograph when 42 years old. The patient worked as a labourer, there was no pain and full movement. Seen 1976, no deterioration (a and c reproduced from Ratliff (1967) by permission of the Editor of J. Bone Jt Surg.)

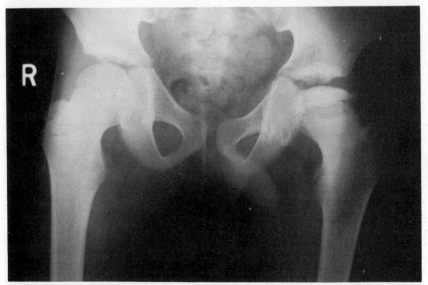

Figure 4.19. Illustrating an unexpected fair result in an older child. (a) Radiograph on admission in 1936 of a boy aged 12 years showing head at risk with lateral subluxation

161

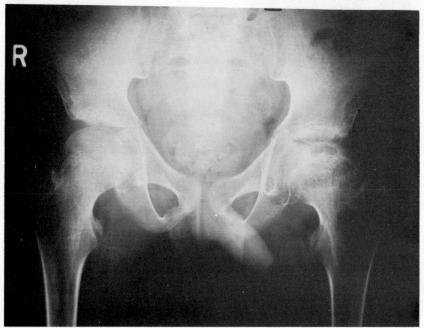

Figure 4.19. (b) Radiograph after 26 months of frame fixation; flattened head incompletely contained

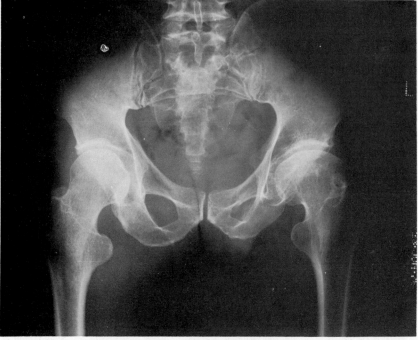

Figure 4.19. (c) Radiograph in 1976 aged 52. Works as a joiner with only minor aches. Incongruous congruity; no deterioration since 1964

pain and had good movements. To illustrate the many factors involved four examples are shown where the head was at risk, two of which were treated and two untreated (*Figures 4.16, 4.17, 4.18* and *4.19*).

Of the various radiological signs described by Catterall of the head at risk, lateral subluxation and lateral encroachment appear to be the most important. This is supported by Kamhi and MacEwen (1975) and Dickens and Menelaus (1976).

4. CONCLUSIONS

(a) A study of 34 cases of Perthes' disease followed for an average of 30 years shows that, while only 2 out of 5 were radiologically normal, no less than 4 out of 5 were fully active and free from pain.

(b) A further study of 16 of these same hips (10 treated, 6 untreated) followed-up for 41 years showed that clinical deterioration rarely occurred and many patients had no pain and normal activity.

(c) Only one-third of these patients had good anatomical results.

(d) There is a characteristic appearance of incongruous congruity in adult life which is compatible with good function up to the age of 50 and perhaps longer.

(e) Where the upper femoral epiphysis remains well contained, either without treatment in mild Perthes' disease or following treatment in severe disease, the long-term result in the adult is likely to be good (*Figure 4.15*).

(f) A limited study suggests that the concept of the 'head at risk' is significant. The two most important signs are lateral subluxation and lateral encroachment. Although the clinical result was often good when the femoral head was not fully covered by the acetabulum at the end of treatment, the radiological result in adult life was never good.

(g) There are many factors to be considered in the prognosis and treatment of Perthes' disease. The debate on the need for treatment or the value of various types of treatment will only be clarified by an analysis of long-term results into adult life. It must be constantly borne in mind that a high proportion of satisfactory clinical results can be achieved with no treatment at all.

Acknowledgement

Despite the apparently endless debate on the aetiology and treatment of Perthes' disease, few long-term studies into adult life are available and the author is grateful to Sir Harry Platt for his unique documentation of a group of children, providing the initial opportunity for this study.

REFERENCES

Brotherton, B. J. and McKibbin, B. (1976). The long-term results of the treatment of Perthes' disease by recumbency and femoral head containment. *J. Bone Jt Surg.* **58B,** 131
Catterall, A. (1971). The natural history of Perthes' disease. *J. Bone Jt Surg.* **53B,** 37

REFERENCES

Catterall, A. (1972). Coxa Plana. *Mod. Trends Orthop.* **6,** 122

Danielsson, L. G. and Hernborg, J. (1965). Late results of Perthes' Disease. *Acta Orthop. Scand.* **36,** 70

Dickens, D. R. V. and Menelaus, M. B. (1976). The assessment of prognosis in Perthes' Disease. *Proc. Combined Mtg Orthop. Ass. English Speaking Wld*

Eaton, G. O. (1967). Long-term results of treatment in coxa plana. *J. Bone Jt Surg.* **49A,** 1031

Gower, W. E. and Johnston, R. C. (1971). Legg–Perthes Disease. *J. Bone Jt Surg.* **53A,** 759

Kamhi, E. and MacEwen, G. D. (1975). The treatment of Legg–Calvé–Perthes Disease. *J. Bone Jt Surg.* **57A,** 651

Lloyd-Roberts, G. C. (1955). Osteoarthritis of Hip. *J. Bone Jt Surg.* **37B,** 8

McKibbin, B. (1975). Recent developments in Perthes' Disease. In *Recent Advances in Orthopaedics,* Edinburgh, London and New York: Churchill Livingstone

Ratliff, A. H. C. (1956). Pseudocoxalgia. *J. Bone Jt Surg.* **38B,** 498

Ratliff, A. H. C. (1967a). Perthes' Disease. A Study of 34 Hips Observed for 30 Years. *J. Bone Jt Surg.* **49B,** 102

Ratliff, A. H. C. (1967b). Osteochondritis dissecans following Legg–Calvé–Perthes Disease. *J. Bone Jt Surg.* **49B,** 108

Salter, R. B., Rang, M., Blackstone, I. W., McArthur, R. C., Weighill, F. J., Cygi, A. C. and Stulberg, S. D. (1976). Perthes' Disease: The scientific basis of methods of management and their indications. *Proc. Combined Mtg Orthop. Ass. English Speaking Wld*

5

Fractures of the Neck of the Femur in Children

A. H. C. Ratliff

A fracture of the neck of the femur in the elderly adult is common, and orthopaedic surgeons have considerable experience in the treatment of this injury and its complications. Conversely, a fracture of the neck of the femur in a child is very rare and in a textbook *'Fractures in Children'* Blount (1955) stated that 'True fractures of the proximal end of the femur are so rare that no one has great experience of them. They are usually indifferently treated with bad results'.

This chapter will summarize the literature and then analyse a study of cases which I have personally made. The author has traced only 8 papers in which more than 20 patients have been studied. Ingram and Bachynski (1953) studied 24 patients treated by the surgeons of the Campbell Clinic, in Memphis, since 1930. They noted that a fracture of the neck of the femur in a child was usually the result of severe trauma, pointing out that avascular necrosis was a serious complication which occurred in 6 out of 17 patients. They advocated treatment of the fracture by internal fixation of the fragments.

McDougall (1961) studied 24 cases collected from a number of surgeons in the West of Scotland. He considered that this injury frequently caused permanent disability; avascular necrosis, non-union, mal-union and disturbance of growth were quite common. Treatment was divided into conservative (immobilization in plaster or traction on a splint) and operative (insertion of a Smith-Petersen pin); McDougall stated that, '. . . equally good or bad results can be obtained by either method' but the numbers cited for each type of treatment were small.

Kite, Lovell and Allman (1962) studied 35 'fractures of the hip' in children. The paper was reported in a few sentences in the Proceedings of the American Orthopaedic Association but no detailed information was given.

Rigault *et al.* (1966) reviewed 25 cases. They stressed the recurrent theme of many authors, namely, the importance and frequency of complications, especially avascular necrosis. They considered treatment to be debatable and advocated conservative management for the transcervical fracture. Lam (1971) reported a study of 75 fractures of the neck of femur in children, aged 8 months to 17 years, seen during a 10-year period (1961–70) in Hong Kong. Despite a large experience he noted that displaced transcervical and cervico-trochanteric fractures, especially if all bone contact had been lost, remained an unsolved problem. He stated that all fractures of the femoral neck in children with the exception of pathological fractures can eventually be made to unite by bone, although bone grafting will sometimes be necessary. The incidence of avascular necrosis in this series was lower than in most previous reports, i.e. 17 per cent in patients seen early. Premature epiphyseal fusion occurred in 17 per cent of patients with fresh fractures. Coxa vara was the commonest complication but it was not incompatible with a good result. In the very young, coxa vara may be modified by remodelling during the process of growth.

Gupta and Chaturvedi (1973) discussed a study of 74 cases below the age of 16 from Kampur in India. Talwalkar (1974) studied 100 cases from Bombay. Gupta stated that displacement osteotomy, both as a primary procedure in transcervical fractures and as a salvage procedure when there are problems of union, gave gratifying results; he stressed the remodelling which can occur at the upper end of the femur with growth. Talwalkar, on the other hand, recommended anatomical reduction and complete immobilization as the treatment of choice in displaced fractures; open reduction should be attempted without hesitation when manipulative reduction was not possible.

Chong Chacha and Lee (1976) described 20 cases from Singapore and in their paper there are 2 cases of acute necrosis of articular cartilage which, as far as I am aware, is the first time this complication has been mentioned after this injury.

CLINICAL MATERIAL

The author first became interested in this injury in 1957 when a boy was admitted to hospital after a double-deck bus toppled on its left side into the basement of a demolished store. Twenty-four patients were admitted to hospital; those who had been on the upper deck of the bus had sustained various important injuries to the left side of the body from direct violence. One of these was a child aged 9 years, suffering from a transcervical fracture of the neck of the left femur. Diagnosis presented no difficulty but very little information was available from senior colleagues or the literature on the best method of treatment.

The principal aim of this chapter is to provide a comprehensive analysis of the natural history and treatment of this injury, occurring in 168 patients (170 fractures). I have treated 30 cases personally, but this was not considered sufficient and therefore an approach was made to the Fellows of the British Orthopaedic Association, a large number of whom kindly permitted me to study the records and radiographs of their cases. The mean period of observation was 5 years, with a minimum of 2 years and a maximum of 25 years. This analysis will be described as the Bristol Study.

Incidence

Allende and Lezama (1951) calculated that for every child who sustained a fracture of the femoral neck there were 300 adults; Peltokallio and Kurkipää (1959) found in Finland that there were 34 fractures in adults to every fracture in a child.

CLINICAL MATERIAL

At an early stage in the Bristol Study a comparison was made between the incidence of fractures of the neck of the femur in children and that in adults admitted to the Manchester Royal Infirmary. In the 12 consecutive years from 1947 to 1959, 7 patients under 17 years of age were admitted to this hospital suffering from fractures of the femoral neck. In the same period about 900 adults were admitted with this injury – a ratio of 1 to 130.

These fractures occurred in children of all ages from 2 to 16 years, the highest incidence being in those aged from 11 to 16 years, inclusive, which accounted for 107 of 168 children. There were 98 boys and 70 girls.

The mechanism of injury

The mechanism of injury in this series of 168 patients is shown in Table 5.I.

TABLE 5.I
The mechanism of injury in 168 patients

Type of injury	Number of patients	Mechanism	
Severe	136	Fall from a height	52
		Knocked over – motor accident	60
		Fall off a bicycle	20
		Fall from a swing	4
Mild	12	Slipped while walking	
		Pushed over	
Miscellaneous	13	–	
Unknown	7	–	

Whilst it was not always easy to assess accurately the severity of injury to which the child was exposed, nevertheless it was considered that the fracture was caused by severe violence in 136 out of 168 patients, i.e. 80 per cent. There were three common types of severe violence: the most frequent was a motor-traffic accident when the child, while walking, was struck by a moving vehicle; the second commonest was a fall from a height – this could include such injuries as falling off a horse, a wall, a tree, a first-floor window or even, as in one case, a 50-foot chimney; and the third commonest type, children who were knocked off scooters or bicycles. The 4 patients who fell from swings landed on concrete. A number of children were involved in accidents in which the precise mechanism was not known and could have been mild or severe. These mechanisms have been described as miscellaneous: examples include a fall in the gym, a fall off a banister rail, and a wall falling on the patient. The child slipping while walking or being pushed over, in only 12 cases, are classified as mild. It is perhaps of some interest that only 2 children sustained this fracture whilst skiing; presumably injuries from this sport produce stress below the neck of the femur.

Experience from India (Gupta, Chaturvedi and Pruthi, 1975) would appear in general to be similar though in that country falling from a height is stressed and occurred in 71 per cent of patients; approximately half of these children fell from trees, mostly during the rainy season. Only 12 per cent sustained a fracture of the neck of the femur by some form of road-traffic accident.

Associated injuries

Sixty-one patients (31 per cent) sustained various other important injuries. The two most commonly associated with a fracture of the neck of the femur were a head injury with a history of concussion (28) and a fracture of the pelvis (12). In 8 patients important multiple injuries occurred necessitating urgent operations or transfusions to save life. The majority of these associated conditions did not prevent treatment of the fracture of the neck of the femur, but in 12 children treatment was delayed for variable periods, seldom for more than three weeks. In 2 cases urgent laparotomy operations were necessary immediately after injury, one because of a ruptured spleen and the other because of a ruptured bladder. Thus, a fracture of the neck of the femur in a child occurs in different circumstances from the common fracture which follows trivial injury in the elderly adult. The child's fracture is not produced easily and severe violence is usually necessary. Indeed, the rarity of this injury compared with other fractures in children would suggest that the neck of the femur in a child is especially strong and resistant to trauma. Two further observations indicate that direct violence on the outer side of the hip, rather than rotation strains, may be required to produce this fracture:

1. In 11 children a fracture of the neck of the femur was associated with a fracture of the superior pubic ramus on the same side. (Fractures of the pubic rami may be due to lateral crushing — Watson-Jones, 1955).
2. In 25 other children severe bruising was recorded in the documents on the lateral side of the hip.

Diagnosis

In this series the diagnosis usually presented no difficulty, and severe violence, marked pain in the region of the hip and an external rotation deformity, drew immediate attention to the possibility of fracture. The diagnosis was confirmed by radiographs. There was delay in diagnosis in 7 children out of a total of 168. The explanation for this delay was as follows:

1. In 3 patients there was only mild disability and the fracture was undisplaced; for example, a girl aged 10 years had fallen off a horse but was able to continue riding and only presented to an orthopaedic surgeon 5 weeks after injury.
2. In another patient there was a fracture of the pelvis, the symptoms were attributed to this injury and a traumatic separation of the upper femoral epiphysis was not noted until 6 weeks after the accident.

3. In 1 patient a traumatic separation of the upper femoral epiphysis was incorrectly diagnosed as a congenital coxa vara.
4. In 2 cases a fracture of the neck of the femur was associated with a fracture of the shaft of the tibia in the same limb and in one of these the diagnosis was tragically missed until some 5 months after injury.

Classification

Fractures of the neck of the femur in children have been classified previously into four types: transepiphyseal, transcervical, cervico-trochanteric and basal, and pertrochanteric. This classification was ascribed originally to Delbet but the reference cannot be traced; it was cited by Colonna and he has been copied in subsequent papers (Ingram and Bachynski, 1953; McDougall, 1961; Kite, Lovell and Allman, 1962; and Ratliff, 1962).

However, the description 'transepiphyseal' is not anatomically correct; the fracture line occurs at the upper femoral epiphyseal plate but does not cross or penetrate the epiphysis of the head of the femur. Therefore, the injury usually described as a transepiphyseal fracture should be more accurately termed a 'traumatic separation' of the upper femoral epiphysis. However, reference to the previous literature is essential and it should therefore be stressed that in subsequent parts of this chapter the terms transepiphyseal fracture and traumatic separation of the upper femoral epiphysis are used to describe the same condition. The distribution of the four types of fractures in the present series is summarized in Table 5.II.

TABLE 5.II
Site and nature of fractures in 167 patients (169 fractures)

	Number of fractures
Traumatic separation of the upper femoral epiphysis	13
Transcervical	88
Cervico-trochanteric or basal	55
Pertrochanteric	13
Displaced	126
Undisplaced	43

(One excluded because the precise site of the fracture was unknown)

It should be explained that traumatic separation of the epiphysis in a young child is very rare (Ratliff, 1968b) and that a pertrochanteric fracture also is rare. It is impossible to distinguish between transcervical and basal or cervico-trochanteric fractures before reduction, and examination of the radiographs after reduction, particularly the lateral view, is essential in order to classify these fractures. In making a decision, the position of the fracture at the inferior aspect of the neck of the femur has been constantly examined. Fractures which are at the mid-portion have been described as transcervical and fractures lower than this, where the neck is becoming broad, as basal.

The most common fracture was transcervical and not, as is usually stated, basal. Displacement occurred in 70 per cent. The direction of a basal fracture was usually at a right-angle to that of the neck of the femur, but the line of a transcervical fracture could vary between the extremes of the horizontal and the vertical.

Fractures in the adolescent resembled those in the adult in radiological appearance except that comminution was rare.

Though this study has shown that the most frequent fracture of the neck of the femur in a child is transcervical, nevertheless the author has gradually formed the impression that the distinction between this fracture and the basal one is of academic interest only since, as will be described later, a distinction between these types of fracture does not significantly influence the high incidence of complications or the methods of treatment which can be employed.

Traumatic displacement of the upper femoral epiphysis in young children

Ratliff (1968b) noted the characteristics of this injury based on a study of 13 cases, and various examples are shown in this paper. Colonna (1929) and Ingram and Bachynski (1953) stressed that this fracture should not be confused with the condition commonly described as slipped upper femoral epiphysis. 'It is an acute traumatic separation of a previously normal epiphysis' – Ingram and Bachynski (1953). These cases occurred in children under 9 years of age, they are very rare, and due to severe violence. Despite these characteristics, McDougall (1961) emphasized that the distinction between this injury and slipped upper femoral epiphysis may be difficult to make in the adolescent. Separation occurred at the epiphyseal plate, and severe posterior displacement is frequent. The fracture line does not penetrate the epiphysis. Premature fusion, avascular necrosis, or non-union (individually or together) occurred in 11 of the 13 patients. This is, therefore, a serious injury which is likely to lead to permanent deformity.

COMPLICATIONS

The major complications include avascular necrosis of the proximal fragment, coxa vara, delayed union and non-union, premature epiphyseal fusion, both at the upper end of the femur and at the epiphyses at the lower end of the femur and upper end of the tibia, and shortening of the leg.

A study of the literature has suggested that in general the incidence of these complications is high (Ingram and Bachynski, 1953; McDougall, 1961; and Rigault et al., 1966). Lam (1971) however, noted that the incidence of avascular necrosis in his series was lower than in most previous reports (17 per cent) and that premature epiphyseal fusion occurred in only 17 per cent of patients with fresh fractures. He considered that coxa vara was the most common complication.

In the Bristol Study one or more complications occurred in 87 of the 126 displaced fractures, i.e. 69 per cent. Complications also occurred even when there was no initial displacement (14 out of 43 cases, i.e. 33 per cent).

COMPLICATIONS

A displaced fracture of the femoral neck is one of the most serious injuries a child can sustain and poor results may show several complications in the same patient and be associated with severe and permanent disability.

AVASCULAR NECROSIS

This is undoubtedly the most important complication. In adults, part or all of the capital fragment may become necrotic but the repair process often comes to a halt before revascularization is completed, leaving a dense zone of fibrous tissue between living and necrotic bone. The segment of necrotic bone eventually collapses under the stress of bearing weight and in the adult this becomes evident clinically some time between the second and third year after injury, and has been described as late segmental collapse (Catto, 1965). In a recent study (Barnes *et al.*, 1976), the incidence of late segmental collapse in the adult was noted to be 24 per cent. Diagnosis may be on clinical grounds (pain and reduced movement) or, more accurately, by histological examination or radiographic evidence. An histological diagnosis was not possible in this study since operative removal of the head of the femur in a child was considered bad treatment and never performed. Radiological diagnosis of avascular necrosis in the child is not precise and is based on the observation of a characteristic increase in density.

Detailed analysis of avascular necrosis after a fracture of the femoral neck in a child is not available in the literature and the aim of this section is to present observations on the incidence, patterns of necrosis, prognosis and treatment of this complication.

Incidence

Avascular necrosis occurred in 78 cases (46 per cent) and it developed in children of all age groups. The effect of age on the incidence is shown in *Figure 5.1*.

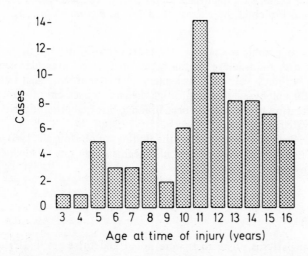

Figure 5.1. The effect of age on incidence of avascular necrosis (78 cases)

The site and nature of the fracture in 78 cases who developed avascular necrosis is shown in Table 5.III.

TABLE 5.III
Site and nature of the fracture in 78 cases where avascular
necrosis developed

	Number of fractures
Traumatic separation of the upper femoral epiphysis	6
Transcervical	50
Basal	20
Pertrochanteric	1
Not known	1

Avascular necrosis occurred in 64 patients in whom the fragments were displaced. Its occurrence in two circumstances is noteworthy:

1. It may follow a basal fracture of the neck of the femur (20 patients) (Ratliff, 1962, Figures 3 and 4). As far as the author is aware, this complication only occurs very rarely, after a similar type of basal fracture in the adult.

2. It may complicate an undisplaced fracture (14 patients), i.e. approximately one-third of all the undisplaced fractures. Apart from a paper by Durbin (1959), this problem is given little emphasis in the literature, and suggests that the diaphyseal vessels may play a more important part in the blood supply of the epiphysis than has been recognized previously. It is important also to give a guarded prognosis after an undisplaced fracture of the neck of the femur in a child. An example is shown in *Figure 5.2 (a), (b)*.

In the adult, radiographic evidence of avascular necrosis may not occur until 2 or more years after the fracture. In this study of children, avascular necrosis always appeared within 1 year after the injury. A frequent early sign was loss of definition of the epiphyseal plate indicating the commencement of premature fusion. This observation has repeatedly been found to be of value in the prediction of the onset of avascular necrosis.

The author has been unable to confirm the findings of McDougall (1961) who stated that the 'radiological signs of avascular necrosis may not be obvious for two years after an injury'.

Patterns of necrosis

Three radiological patterns of necrosis were noted and these are illustrated in *Figure 5.3*.

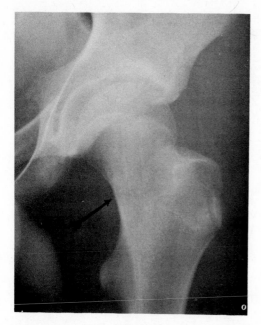

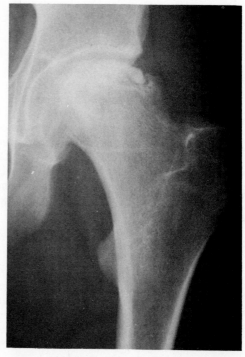

Figure 5.2. (a) An example of an undisplaced fracture in a boy aged 16 who was knocked off a bicycle

Figure 5.2. (b) Radiograph of the same hip 1 year later showing severe diffuse necrosis

Type of necrosis

I   II   III

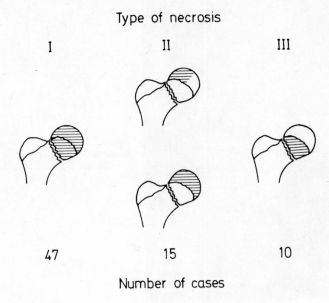

47   15   10

Number of cases

*Figure 5.3. Diagram to illustrate the three radiological types
of avascular necrosis*

Type I

In this type the avascular necrosis was diffuse and involved the entire fragment of
bone including the epiphysis proximal to the fracture line. This pattern was the
most frequent and occurred in 47 cases. The radiographic features were similar
to those commonly observed after a fracture of the femoral neck in the adult.
Necrosis of bone was accompanied by various degrees of collapse of the proximal
fragment. In some patients, severe diffuse collapse occurred followed by subluxation of the hip; in others, segmental necrosis was largely confined to part
of the head of the femur. In another group of patients, no significant collapse
developed but the femoral head later showed a curious coarse trabecular appearance. The explanation of these changes is not known but it is presumed that
they are the result of revascularization. Examples of these various types of
necrosis are shown in *Figures 5.4 (a)* and *(b)*.

Type II

In 15 patients avascular changes were apparently confined to the epiphysis and
the femoral neck distal to the epiphyseal plate appeared normal. An increase in
density occasionally affected part of the epiphysis but was more commonly
diffuse and involved the whole of the epiphysis. An example illustrating these
changes is shown in *Figure 5.5*.

174

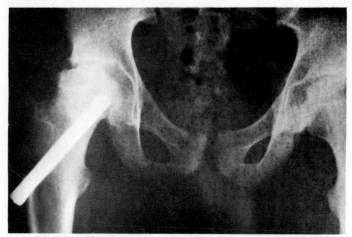

Figure 5.4. (a) To illustrate Type I severe diffuse necrosis. The right hip of a boy, aged 15 years, 18 months after a transcervical fracture. The fracture has united. Later arthrodesis necessary

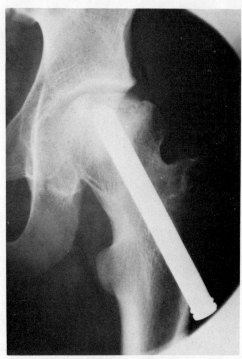

Figure 5.4. (b) To illustrate Type I necrosis with segmental collapse. The left hip of a boy aged 16, 1 year after a transcervical fracture with marked displacement. Despite these appearances symptoms were slight and he played football

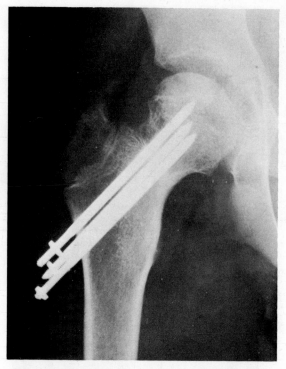

Figure 5.5. Radiograph demonstrating a united fracture 7 months after injury with revascularization of the upper femoral epiphysis. Early premature fusion. Fragmentation never occurred. An example of Type II necrosis

Type III

In this group the necrosis occurred in 10 patients and the changes appeared to be confined to the femoral neck and produced a radiographic appearance which was first mentioned by McDougall in 1961 and independently described by the author (1962).

On examining previous case reports, the author has observed radiographs illustrating avascular necrosis of the femoral neck though these radiographs have been published without comment on this condition (Carrell and Carrell, 1941; Allende and Lezama, 1951; Lam, 1964 and 1965). In the author's series 11 patients showed uniform increase in density which appeared in the femoral neck shortly after the fracture occurred, accurately outlined proximally by the epiphyseal plate and distally by the fracture line. The capital epiphysis appeared less dense than the femoral neck and did not collapse or fragment, though it sometimes later demonstrated a coarse, trabecular appearance. There was a striking incidence of premature fusion at the upper femoral epiphyseal plate which occurred in 6 out of 11 patients with this type of necrosis. The work of Harris and Bobechko (1960) suggests that the radiographic appearance of

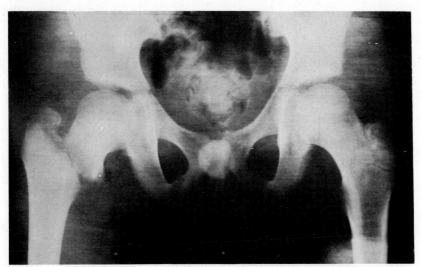

Figure 5.6. To illustrate Type III necrosis. (a) Radiograph of a child aged 11 shortly after injury

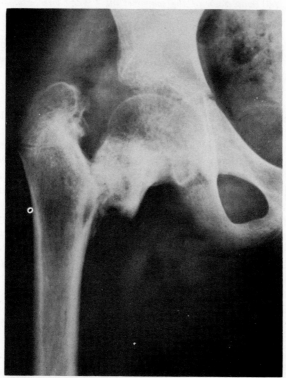

Figure 5.6. (b) Radiograph 5 months later showing increased density of the femoral neck. The epiphysis is less dense but not flattened or fragmented

177

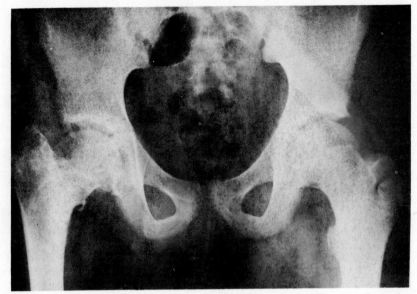

Figure 5.6. (c) Radiograph of the same patient 4 years later. Premature fusion has occurred

Type III necrosis indicates new bone formation laid down on bone which has become avascular since the injury. An example of avascular necrosis of the femoral neck Type III is shown in *Figure 5.6 (a), (b)* and *(c)*.

The relationship of avascular necrosis after a fracture to Perthes' disease

In order to compare these two conditions a study has been made of 18 patients who developed avascular necrosis after a fracture (Ratliff, 1968). These 18 cases were chosen as their ages were between 5 and 10 years at the time of injury and therefore in the age group most likely to develop appearances characteristic of Perthes' disease. Such changes occurred in only 1 patient and this patient was only observed for a short period of 4 months. It may be concluded that the radiological appearances of avascular necrosis after a fracture of the femoral neck in a child are different from the cycle of changes accepted as those of Perthes' disease. These facts offer new evidence that Perthes' disease is not simply avascular necrosis due to damage to the arterial blood supply of the upper end of the neck and head of the femur.

Prognosis

The prognosis of avascular necrosis is illustrated in Table 5.IV.

It was particularly significant that no good results were obtained with Type I necrosis. Occasionally revascularization did develop after Type II or III necrosis. Thus, this complication usually affected the prognosis adversely, though there

TABLE 5.IV
The prognosis of avascular necrosis in 72 cases

Result	Type I	Type II	Type III	Totals
Good	–	3	3	6
Fair	12	7	7	26
Poor	35	4	1	40

were some notable exceptions. No evidence could be found to suggest that avascular necrosis was related to the direction of the fracture line, any one mechanism of injury, or any one method of treatment. The author has analysed these cases carefully but could find no really convincing evidence of any case of cartilage necrosis in this series.

Treatment

It will be appreciated that in many of these children several complications occurred and in this section it is proposed to consider the treatment of avascular necrosis where delayed union or non-union did not develop.

Type I

When a child develops this complication he may present with either mild or severe symptoms though the radiological characteristics are obvious.

In 25 children where the symptoms were mild, the child was either given no treatment or a weight-relieving caliper. The results of treatment in these 25 patients were classified as 21 fair and 4 poor. There were important changes visible in the radiographs though the child usually had slight complaints and the hips showed good movements. The period of observation in some of these cases was short and the ultimate fate of the hip joint not known. Many of these children had a tolerable hip for the period of observation but are likely to develop osteoarthritis of the joint in the years to come and may require surgical treatment in early adult life.

When symptoms are severe, often with subluxation of the hip joint, the only treatment which would appear to be of value is an arthrodesis (performed in 6 children). It is perhaps of some interest to note that 8 children had a subtrochanteric osteotomy performed in the hope that this operation might improve the blood supply to the head and neck of the femur, but the author was not convinced that the process of revascularization was materially affected by this operation and all 8 cases had poor results at the time of review.

With the tremendous changes in the attitude to hip surgery in the last 5 to 10 years, it is possible that many of these children may in early adult life present with severe symptoms and then a difficult decision will have to be made as to whether an arthrodesis or the more topical total hip replacement should be performed. No experience can be recorded on this subject from this study.

It should also be noted that a muscle pedicle transplant bone-grafting operation has recently been used in the treatment of displaced transcervical fractures in the adult (Meyers, Harvey and Moore, 1973) but, again, there is no record of this operation having been performed in any fractures of the neck of the femur in children. It would appear to the author to be a reasonable approach to what is otherwise a very difficult and unsolved problem.

Type II

Only 4 patients were given treatment for this complication and therefore no precise conclusions can be given. The x-ray changes were dissimilar to those characteristic of Perthes' disease and the best treatment is not known.

Type III

There were 10 patients who showed evidence of necrosis localized to the femoral neck but only 1 was given treatment for this condition, namely a weight-relieving caliper for a period of 9 months. The author has gained the impression that this type of necrosis is the least important since revascularization always occurs without collapse of the femoral neck. Treatment is probably unnecessary and this type of necrosis is of academic interest only. However, it has already been shown that it may be associated with premature fusion of the upper femoral epiphyseal plate leading to a deformity; this further complication cannot be prevented but may require treatment in later life. An example is shown in *Figure 5.6 (a), (b)* and *(c)*.

DELAYED UNION AND NON-UNION

Delayed union is an arbitrary term which cannot be defined precisely and has been applied to cases where radiographic evidence of union was not present 5 months after injury, but where union later occurred without surgical treatment.

Non-union after a fracture in a child is a very rare problem and the occurrence of non-union after a fracture of the neck of the femur was questioned by Colonna (1929) and Mitchell (1936). Lam (1971) stated that in his study of 75 fractures with early open reduction and sometimes bone grafting all the fractures in his series ultimately united. Non-union occurred in 4 of the late fractures. In 3 of the latter the non-union was probably associated with delay in diagnosis.

In a series of 24 patients described by Ingram and Bachynski (1953) there was 1 case of non-union, and there were 2 cases of non-union in McDougall's series of 24 patients.

In this Bristol Study delayed union was present in some 22 cases and non-union developed in a further 17 out of a total of 126 displaced fractures. Difficulties of union therefore occurred in 31 per cent, i.e. approximately one-third of all the cases of displaced fractures. No fracture which was undisplaced at the time of injury developed non-union. There would appear to be a number of causes for non-union in the 17 cases in this study. Union failed in 5 patients

where displaced fractures were treated by manipulative reduction and immobilization of the hip in a plaster spica; in 2 an adequate reduction was not
achieved and in 3 displacement of the fragments recurred. An important single
cause of non-union was the acceptance of the displaced position of the fragments
and immobilization in a hip spica.

Another important cause of non-union is unsatisfactory internal fixation,
either because reduction was poor, internal fixation inadequate, or the fragments
left distracted. These problems occurred in 5 patients. Union failed in 4 patients
with severe multiple injuries where satisfactory initial treatment of the fracture
could not be carried out and in 1 case where the fracture was missed for 5 months
due to other injuries of the same limb.

Finally, non-union occurred in 1 patient after a primary osteotomy and in
1 patient after a satisfactory primary internal fixation. It should be noted that
all these were very difficult problems, that avascular necrosis occurred as well as
non-union in 7 of the 17 patients and only 6 eventually obtained a good result
after various types of salvage procedure. Permanent non-union was established
in 8 patients. It is concluded that every endeavour must be made to prevent the
occurrence of this very serious complication. Accurate reduction of the fragments
of the fracture is necessary and internal fixation required. The author now
believes that, when necessary, open reduction should be performed. A short
delay in beginning treatment did not have an adverse effect on union, providing
adequate reduction was achieved and maintained; even in those cases with
multiple injuries it may be that a bolder approach is necessary in order to
prevent this serious complication.

The treatment of non-union after a fracture in a child is difficult. Clearly
each case has to be considered on its merits but it should be noted that in 5
children good results were obtained after a bone-grafting operation, usually a
fibula graft inserted up the neck of the femur, and also with internal fixation.
An aggressive approach should be adopted since the disability with permanent
non-union is high. An illustrative case is shown in *Figure 5.7 (a)* and *(b)*. If
severe coxa vara is present in addition to the non-union, particularly in younger
children, then an abduction osteotomy should be performed.

COXA VARA

In the adult femur the neck is set on the shaft at an angle which varies from
120° to 140° (Mercer and Duthie, 1964). A decrease in this neck-shaft angle
results in mechanical disadvantages; the great trochanter is displaced upwards,
there is shortening of the leg and a marked Trendelenburg limp. McDougall
(1961) and Imhäuser (1963) stated that there was a marked tendency to coxa
vara after a fracture of the femoral neck in childhood. Strange (1965) considered
that the varus may even be so acute that the angle between the neck and the
shaft is reduced to less than 90°. Any further growth in the capital epiphyseal
plate then pushes the trochanteric end of the femur upwards and actually
progressively increases the shortening. Lam (1971) stated that coxa vara was the
commonest complication (32 per cent) in his study, but he stressed that this
was not incompatible with a good result; in the very young the coxa vara may be
modified by remodelling during the process of growth. The general impression

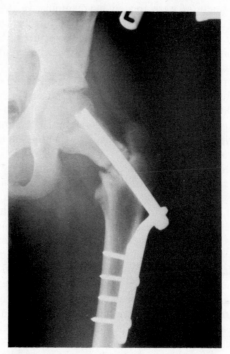

Figure 5.7. To illustrate the successful treatment of non-union. (a) Radiograph of a boy aged 14 with non-union 5 months after a basal fracture of the neck of the femur

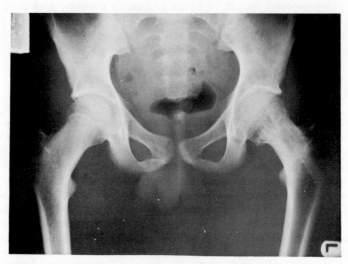

Figure 5.7. (b) Radiograph of the same patient 15 months later after a fibular graft had been inserted with also an iliac bone graft laid on the front of the fracture. Bony union with excellent function

is gained from the literature that coxa vara is associated with delayed or non-union, particularly when the fracture is immobilized in a plaster spica and that with internal fixation of the fragments 'its incidence is reduced to a minimum'

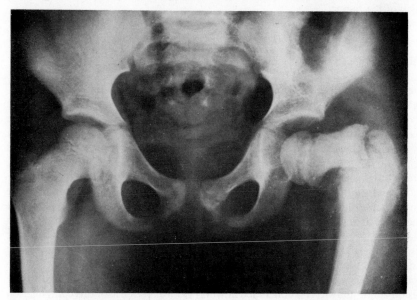

Figure 5.8. An example of a basal fracture with a severe coxa vara deformity in a child aged 6, 1 month after injury. This deformity must never be accepted

(Ingram and Bachynski, 1953). Coxa vara occurred in 26 patients in the Bristol Study (15 per cent) and may be associated with delayed or non-union. An example is shown in *Figure 5.8*.

The deformity occurred in several circumstances:

1. When early treatment of the fracture of the femur was not possible because of the presence of multiple injuries.
2. When the fracture was either not reduced or the fragments became displaced after manipulative reduction and immobilization in a plaster spica.
3. Rarely, when union of the fracture after a subtrochanteric osteotomy appeared adequate but an adduction deformity later developed between the neck and shaft of the femur.

Coxa vara should be prevented and it is noteworthy in the Bristol Study that it did not occur when adequate primary fixation had been achieved. The treatment of coxa vara is debatable because of the alterations which occur in the shape of the upper end of the femur with growth. The author agrees with Lam that remodelling of the upper end of the femur often occurs, particularly in younger children, and that it may be corrected to a large extent with growth. Providing union of the fracture has occurred a mild degree of coxa vara usually requires no treatment. However, when the angle between the neck and the shaft of the femur is less than 90°, remodelling cannot occur and an abduction osteotomy is essential. Displacement of the distal fragment under the neck of the femur is not necessary and it would prevent remodelling with progressive growth of the neck of the femur.

PREMATURE EPIPHYSEAL FUSION

Premature fusion at the upper femoral epiphyseal plate was a frequent complication; it occurred in 43 cases and accompanied the three types of necrosis. In Type I necrosis, where the changes were diffuse and severe, premature fusion was relatively unimportant compared with the partial or total collapse of the head of the femur and subluxation of the hip joint. However, in patients in whom the upper femoral epiphysis did not collapse, especially if the child was young, premature fusion was an important complication and the cause of late deformity.

Premature fusion also occurred in one or both epiphyseal plates of the knee on the same side as the fracture in 6 patients, resulting in shortening which, at the time of review, varied from 1½ to 3½ in (40–90 mm). This complication developed in 4 of these 6 children after prolonged immobilization, often after secondary salvage operations because of complications of treatment of the original fracture. With one exception there was no evidence of any injury to the epiphyseal plate at the lower end of the femur and the precise cause of premature fusion is not known. It is concluded however from experience of this complication in other conditions, that every attempt must be made to avoid the need for prolonged immobilization and secondary salvage operations.

SHORTENING

Shortening of the leg after a fracture of the neck of the femur in a child is, perhaps not surprisingly, a frequent complication and it was recorded in 54 patients in this study, varying from as little as ½ in (15 mm) to as much as 5 in (130 mm). As the period of observation of these growing children was variable, a detailed analysis of the amount of shortening has not been made. The causes of this shortening may be briefly summarized.

1. Avascular necrosis of the head of the femur. When the necrosis was severe with diffuse collapse, subluxation of the hip occurred.
2. Avascular necrosis with premature fusion at the upper femoral epiphyseal plate. Premature fusion was always associated with avascular necrosis except in 3 cases of traumatic separation of the upper femoral epiphysis. No explanation can be given as to why premature fusion occurred in some cases of avascular necrosis and not in others, but it may be related to the degree of destruction of the blood supply.
3. Coxa vara.
4. Non-union. This was usually associated with shortening of the neck of the femur itself and thus led to shortening of the limb.
5. Premature fusion at the epiphyses of the knee.

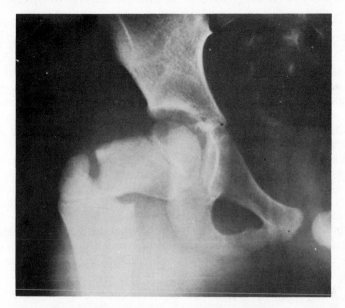

Figure 5.9. (a) Girl aged 8 years, basal fracture of right femoral neck with varus deformity. Manipulative reduction, fragments slipped in plaster, open reduction, internal fixation

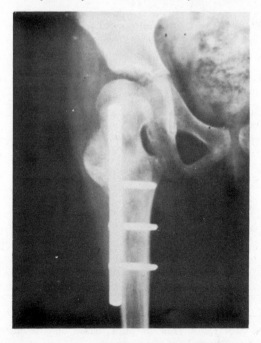

Figure 5.9. (b) Radiograph 8 months after injury, union with coxa valga deformity. Later serious subluxation occurred

185

MISCELLANEOUS COMPLICATIONS

Three other complications occurred which seriously affected the result of treatment and these will be briefly mentioned without detailed discussion.

In one child with a basal fracture with gross displacement, a sciatic nerve palsy occurred and some permanent paresis remained.

In another child, septicaemia due to a salmonella infection occurred immediately after the accident and suppurative arthritis of the injured hip joint followed. The head and neck of the femur were destroyed and an arthrodesis was performed 6 months after injury.

Finally, in a child aged 8 years, an open reduction of a basal fracture was performed three months after an injury which was followed by delayed union and varus deformity. Unfortunately the fracture was internally fixed in a position of coxa valga and 4 years later there was subluxation of the head of the femur and the result was classified as poor *Figure 5.9 (a)* and *(b)*.

It is the author's impression that, no matter what the cause, the deformity of coxa valga in a child never becomes less with growth and this demonstrates the importance of not fixing a fracture of the neck of the femur in this valgus position.

TREATMENT

Classification of results

Results of treatment for various conditions of the hip in childhood are difficult to assess, for it is a common experience to see a patient with no complaints and hips with full movement despite an abnormal radiograph. In this study, results

TABLE 5.V
The assessment of results of treatment

	Good	*Fair*	*Poor*
Pain	None or 'ignores'	Occasional	Severe
Movement	Full or terminal restriction	Greater than 50%	Less than 50%
Activity	Normal	Normal or avoids games	Restricted
Radiographic indications	Normal or mild deformity of the femoral neck	Severe deformity of the femoral neck. 'Mild avascular necrosis'	Severe avascular necrosis. Degenerative arthritis. Arthrodesis

have been classified as good, fair or poor, based on assessment of both the clinical state and the radiographic appearance.

Clinical features such as pain, movement and activity have been noted but particular emphasis has been laid on the radiographic appearance in the belief that this gives an important indication of the likely ultimate prognosis. A summary of the method of assessment of results is given in Table 5.V.

In practice, the result was always classified as good when the fracture united without complications, and as poor where serious complications developed and the function of the hip was certain to be permanently impaired.

Undisplaced fractures

There is little information in the literature concerning the treatment of undisplaced fractures of the neck of the femur in a child. Lam (1971) stated that undisplaced or minimally displaced fresh fractures of the neck of the femur in children carried a good prognosis and that simple methods of treatment were no less effective in these patients than were operative measures. No complications occurred and he recommended that this type of fracture should be treated by simple immobilization in a plaster spica for a period of 6 weeks, or perhaps in an older child a little longer.

Avascular necrosis can follow an undisplaced fracture and 3 cases were described by Durbin (1959).

A number of methods of treatment were employed in the management of 43 undisplaced fractures in this study, the commonest being a plaster spica (20), and internal fixation (6); other methods included the use of a Thomas splint, bed-rest, skin traction, frame fixation and, in one case, no treatment at all. In 32 patients a good result was obtained although in 2 of these mild avascular necrosis occurred (later the upper femoral epiphysis revascularized). Of the 7 patients who obtained a fair result, 5 developed avascular necrosis without collapse of the upper femoral epiphysis. In 1 patient displacement of the fragments occurred 3 weeks after injury whilst the hip was immobilized in a plaster spica and delayed union with mild avascular necrosis developed requiring a bone-grafting operation. In the other patient the fragments became displaced while the patient was resting in bed and open reduction with internal fixation was necessary 5 weeks after injury. Severe avascular necrosis developed in the 4 patients who obtained poor results and the radiographs of 3 of these were published by Durbin (1959).

A more recent and arresting example is shown in *Figure 5.2 (a)* and *(b)*. It appears from the Bristol Study of 43 undisplaced fractures that good results are to be expected with any sound method of conservative care and the author agrees with Lam that probably the best method of treatment is immobilization in a plaster spica in abduction in order to prevent the risk of coxa vara. However, avascular necrosis was an important complication which developed in approximately one-third of the cases of undisplaced fractures and the author agrees with Durbin that for this reason the prognosis should be guarded.

Displacement occurred during the conservative treatment of 2 patients with fractures that had previously been classified as undisplaced. This complication is well recognized following a fracture of the neck of the femur in the adult but has not been described previously in a child. It could be prevented by internal fixation of all undisplaced fractures, but the author does not consider that this operation is merited when the fragments slipped in only 2 out of 43 patients.

Displaced fractures

In sharp contrast, the management of a displaced transcervical fracture or basal fracture in a child, especially if all bone contact has been lost, remains an unsolved problem (Lam, 1971) and frequently results in permanent disability. In the literature, references to treatment are usually short statements based on a study of a relatively small number of cases and the opinions expressed about the value of different methods of treatment are conflicting. No reference can be found to any comparison of the types of primary treatment or results of salvage operations which may be necessary in these difficult cases. This section will discuss the treatment of 126 displaced fractures.

Primary treatment

This term has been used to indicate the major treatment during the first 3 weeks after injury. A good result was obtained in only 40 cases, almost exactly one-third. In a further 12 patients a good result was eventually achieved after a secondary salvage procedure. A number of methods of treatment were employed in the management of these patients and these will be discussed.

TABLE 5.VI
The primary treatment of displaced fractures*

Primary treatment	Number of fractures	Number of good results
Manipulation and plaster spica	37	7
Manipulation and internal fixation	52	21
Manipulative reduction, internal fixation and bone graft	2	1
Subtrochanteric osteotomy	6	2
Manipulative reduction with skeletal or skin traction	6	3
Open reduction and internal fixation	12	4
Manipulation and Thomas splint	3	1
None	8	1
Totals	126	40

* 125 patients, 1 bilateral

Manipulative reduction and immobilization in a plaster spica

This method was employed in 37 patients. In 23 the fracture was either not accurately reduced or the fragments became displaced after reduction. In 6 other patients a good position was maintained but avascular necrosis occurred and only 7 children obtained a good result after primary treatment by this method.

The author has the impression that if other methods had been used, particularly with the older adolescent children, then the results of treatment in this study as a whole would have been improved. For these reasons manipulative reduction and immobilization in a plaster spica as the treatment of choice for displaced fractures is not recommended. Lam (1971) however, considers that an attempt at closed reduction is a reasonable step and then advocates the application of a plaster spica in the younger patients; but he recommends in an older child the use of internal fixation and application of a plaster spica.

Manipulative reduction and internal fixation

This was the commonest procedure for the primary treatment of displaced fractures. It was carried out in 52 patients, the majority of whom (39) had transcervical fractures, though 10 were basal and 3 intertrochanteric. Many types of internal fixation were used including Smith-Petersen pins (most frequent) and smaller pins such as those of Moore, Newman or Knowle.

In this series, distraction of the fragments produced by insertion of a Smith-Petersen or similar large trifin pin occurred in 10 patients; this led to difficulties during the operation and was one of the causes of delay in union. For this reason a three-flanged nail or pin of any type should not be used and smaller pins are preferred. Some surgeons have been careful when inserting the pin to avoid crossing the epiphyseal plate because it was feared that penetration of the plate might result in premature epiphyseal fusion. In this study a careful analysis was made concerning this particular aspect; premature fusion of the upper end of the femur was always associated with avascular necrosis and there were no cases in which premature fusion could be attributed to a pin crossing the epiphyseal plate in the absence of avascular necrosis. The author was unable to confirm the conclusions of McDougall that internal fixation is contra-indicated because it may cause necrosis and damage to the epiphysis.

The following conclusions are drawn from this study:

1. Of those patients treated by manipulative reduction and internal fixation (52) less than one-half obtained a good result (21). A growing impression is developing that an accurate reduction is essential, particularly in the transcervical type of fracture in the adolescent child, and that unless a good reduction is obtained with adequate fixation complications are likely to develop (*Figure 5.10 (a)* and *(b)*).

   It will be noted that the percentage of good results following manipulative reduction and internal fixation in these fractures in children is much lower than for a similar problem in, for example, an elderly lady.

2. There were 5 cases of non-union and these were attributed to poor reduction or inadequate fixation. Non-union and serious mal-union with coxa vara were prevented by internal fixation providing that the method was technically adequate. These observations support those of Ingram and Bachynski, and of Imhauser who considered that one of the important advantages of internal fixation was the prevention of non-union and coxa vara.

189

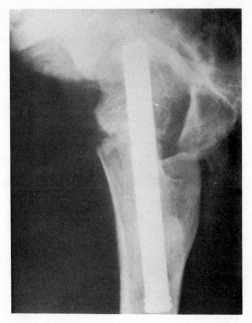

Figure 5.10. Never accept a bad reduction. Arthrodesis later necessary. (a) Position immediately after internal fixation

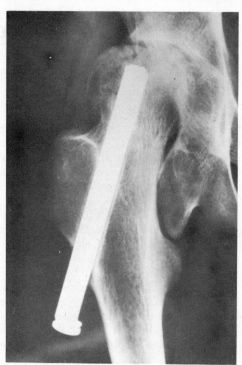

Figure 5.10. (b) Radiographs 10 months later. The hip is subluxated with severe avascular necrosis

3. Poor results were due to avascular necrosis and, in a small number of cases, non-union also occurred. Avascular necrosis was not predictable except when a poor reduction of the fracture had occasionally been accepted; it was always associated with severe necrosis Type I and a poor result.

Subtrochanteric osteotomy

This is a well recognized operation for the treatment of non-union of a fracture of the neck of the femur in the adult. 'The purpose of an abduction osteotomy is to turn the shaft from the adducted to the abducted position so that the shearing stress of weight-bearing and muscle retraction becomes an impaction force' (Watson-Jones, 1955). Recently it has been advocated in the primary treatment of intracapsular fractures in the adult. The operation has been used for cases in which the risk of non-union is increased, such as when there is a 'steep' fracture line, marked comminution, or failure to reduce the displacement by manipulation.

Primary subtrochanteric osteotomy was performed in 6 patients in this series because of failure to obtain a good position with manipulative reduction. Four of these 6 children obtained a reasonable result; the 2 poor results were due, in one patient, to severe avascular necrosis and, in the other, to non-union of the fracture despite osteotomy.

There are several conclusions to be drawn from this small series:

1. Remarkable remodelling of the upper end of the femur with growth may occur after osteotomy. This was noteworthy when the osteotomy was low and when a gap was left between the inferior part of the neck of the femur and the upper part of the distal fragment. Remodelling cannot occur if the distal fragment is placed close under the neck of the femur, and in these cases shortening may result.
2. Late varus may develop at the site of the osteotomy, even after union. The tendency to varus should be anticipated when performing this operation and the distal fragment should be deliberately placed in marked abduction.
3. Primary osteotomy is a useful procedure which may have to be performed when manipulative reduction has not been successful.

Gupta, Chaturvedi and Pruthi (1975) stressed the use of primary osteotomy in a large series of cases (135) and stated that 71 per cent obtained good results with a transcervical fracture. They also stressed the considerable remodelling that can occur at the upper end of the femur after this operation. No other reference can be found to this method of treatment in the literature.

Reduction with skeletal or skin traction

This method was employed in 6 patients; 4 of these obtained a good result. Reduction with traction is particularly suitable for young children with slight displacement, where it is important to maintain the leg in abduction and prevent coxa vara. In my opinion it should never be used for the adolescent child with a severely displaced transcervical fracture since it is essential that accurate reduction be achieved and maintained.

Open reduction and internal fixation

At the present time, open reduction of a displaced fracture of the neck of the femur in the adult is seldom employed in Britain. The operation is difficult, the blood supply of the head of the femur may be endangered, and the results are stated to be poor (Green, 1960).

In this study of children, open reduction and internal fixation was performed in 12 cases within the first three weeks after injury. The operation was indicated in the following circumstances:

1. When the displacement was severe and the surgeon considered that manipulative reduction would be of no value.
2. When manipulative reduction had failed.
3. When there were other injuries to the same limb which made other methods of treatment difficult.

Avascular necrosis and non-union were the cause of poor results and only 4 good results were achieved. Thus it is difficult to draw any precise conclusions, for this operation is certainly not easy and there is always the risk of further endangering the blood supply to the proximal fragment. However, with increasing experience, the author is gaining the impression that a more aggressive attitude should be adopted to these severely displaced fractures, particularly in the adolescent child. It is essential to obtain and maintain good reduction, and open reduction may have to be carried out to achieve this object.

Secondary treatment

The need for secondary treatment should be avoided if at all possible. Once complications have developed, even surgeons with considerable experience are faced with a formidable and sometimes insoluble problem. It is not proposed in this section to discuss in detail the further, and often complicated, operations of a salvage nature which were necessary after failure of primary treatment. It is, however, to be noted that such salvage operations were required in 53 patients with displaced fractures (41 per cent). Many different types of operation were carried out and in 10 cases more than one operation was performed. Of these salvage operations the most common was a late subtrochanteric osteotomy (19 cases), further internal fixation coupled with a bone-grafting procedure (8 cases), and an arthrodesis (6 cases). Two observations may be made concerning these salvage operations.

1. Late subtrochanteric osteotomy was a valuable procedure in the management of some difficult cases. In 14 cases, reasonable results were obtained (5 good and 9 fair); with 2 exceptions both the osteotomy and the fracture united and further treatment was not required during the period of observation, though it might well be necessary in later life (*Figure 5.11 (a), (b)* and *(c)*.

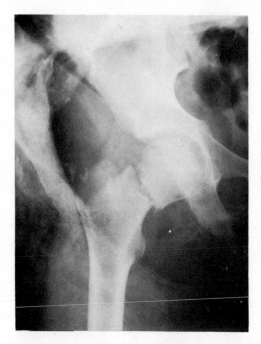

Figure 5.11. To illustrate the value of late subtrochanteric osteotomy. (a) Radiograph of a girl aged 11 after manipulative reduction and immobilization in a hip spica

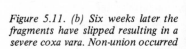

Figure 5.11. (b) Six weeks later the fragments have slipped resulting in a severe coxa vara. Non-union occurred

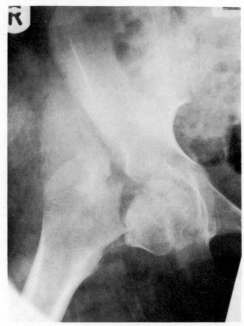

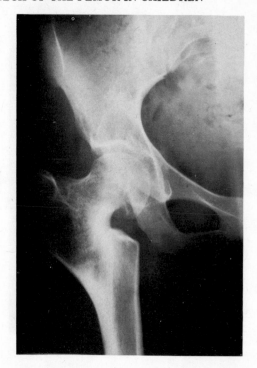

Figure 5.11. (c) Radiograph 4 years later with union and remodelling at the site of the osteotomy

2. Osteotomy was of no value when carried out for avascular necrosis. The operation was performed in some cases, presumably in an endeavour to improve the blood supply of the head of the femur, but the author was not convinced that the cycle of changes was materially affected by this operation and all the results were poor.

When there is severe avascular necrosis with symptoms and growth is fully achieved in early adult life, then the surgeon has a very difficult decision to decide on the relative merits of arthrodesis versus the more modern types of total hip replacement.

No child in this series had a total hip replacement, as far as the author is aware, but no doubt this is a possibility to be considered in the years to come.

Discussion of treatment of displaced fractures

This chapter reports the results of treatment of a rare fracture by many surgeons, and the deficiencies of this method of study are appreciated. Nevertheless, it would appear to be the only method of analysis available. These cases have caused considerable interest to the surgeons responsible for their care. The quality of documentation and radiographs has usually been excellent. The outstanding conclusions to be drawn from this study are that there is a high incidence of serious complications after a fracture of the neck of the femur in the child and that the poor results are due to these complications. Indeed, it should be noted that the incidence of complications is much higher in this study than reported elsewhere. No explanation can be offered for this conclusion but it should be pointed out that no attempt has been made in any way to select the cases and all possible have been included.

The most important complication is severe diffuse avascular necrosis. As far as is known, this cannot be predicted or prevented. However, other complications, such as coxa vara, delayed union or non-union, and growth disturbance at the knee, can often be prevented. A surgeon faced with the difficult problems of a displaced fracture must choose the plan of treatment that is least likely to result in these complications.

Whenever possible, manipulative reduction of a displaced fracture and internal fixation should be carried out. Provided a good reduction can be obtained and internal fixation is adequate, non-union and serious mal-union with a coxa vara deformity are prevented. However, this method only offers a 50 per cent chance of a good result. Poor results are due to avascular necrosis. In my opinion, the fracture should always be immobilized using small pins of the Moore, Newman or Knowle type; because of the danger of distraction, a Smith-Petersen pin should never be used.

If a displaced fracture of the neck of the femur cannot be reduced by manipulation, there are two alternative methods of treatment, namely, primary subtrochanteric osteotomy or open reduction and internal fixation. The evidence provides no precise guidance, since the numbers treated by each method are small. Primary subtrochanteric osteotomy has the advantage of being an easy operation with a good chance of a reasonable result, since remodelling of the upper end of the femur tends to restore normal anatomy. In support of the use of the osteotomy, it may be noted that this was the most frequent salvage operation performed in instances of failure of primary treatment, and it was a valuable procedure in the management of some of these problems. Internal fixation of the subtrochanteric osteotomy was used in 3 patients, but it would appear that this prevented remodelling, and, indeed, fixation in a bad position may in itself lead to a poor result. The best results of osteotomy were obtained when internal fixation was not employed, when the displacement was slight and the lower fragment was placed in wide abduction. There was no evidence that osteotomy was of value when carried out as a salvage procedure for avascular necrosis.

Open reduction and internal fixation aim to restore the normal anatomy and are indicated for fractures where a manipulative reduction has not been successful or is unlikely to succeed. It is especially indicated when the fracture is pertrochanteric and exposure therefore relatively easy. On the other hand, for the transcervical fracture which is displaced, open reduction is difficult. An impression is now being gained that if the operator is experienced, open reduction should be carried out, difficult though it may be; but it is clear from the analysis that no more precise statement can be made at the present time.

In conclusion, the author considers that the major principle in the management of these displaced fractures is that good reduction must be achieved and maintained soon after injury. It is hoped that the universal adoption of this principle in the future will reduce the incidence of some of the serious complications and improve the results of treatment in this major injury.

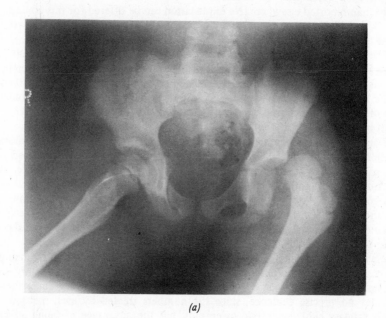

(a)

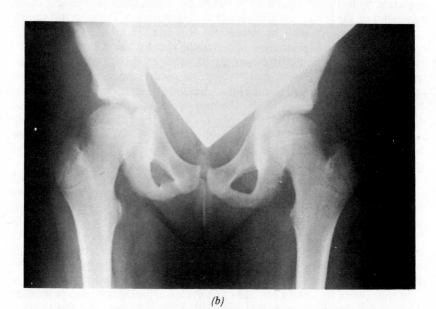

(b)

Figure 5.12. (a) A posterior dislocation of the left hip in a girl aged 4. She had slipped on uneven ground. The leg is adducted and internally rotated. (b) Radiographs 4 years later. A normal hip

196

TRAUMATIC DISLOCATION OF THE HIP IN CHILDREN

This is a rare injury. Glass and Powell (1961) studied the documents of 47 children available for review from a large number of orthopaedic surgeons. The author has seen 3 cases in the last ten years (*Figure 5.12*).

Several well documented reports on this subject have appeared in the literature (Freeman, Jr, 1961; Funk, Jr. 1962; Haliburton, Brockenshire and Barber, 1961; Morton, 1959; Pearson and Mann, 1973; Pennsylvania Orthopaedic Society, 1968; Piggot, 1961; and Wilson, 1966).

This dislocation may occur in children of all age groups. It is more common in males than females. The mechanism of injury is variable. The injury usually responsible is often trivial such as 'doing the splits, slipping on ice, or tripping over in the school playground while walking' (Glass and Powell, 1961). More rarely, especially in older children, dislocation is due to severe violence such as athletic injuries, falls from a height, or as a passenger in a motor traffic accident.

The dislocation is usually posterior, though anterior and central dislocations have been described. No anatomical predisposition has been observed. Rarely, there may be associated fractures of the acetabulum or femoral head (Piggot, 1961). A posterior dislocation produces a flexed adducted and internally rotated leg.

Treatment

Immediate reduction under general anaesthetic by closed methods is essential. A posterior dislocation is reduced by flexing the hip and the knee to 90° and applying traction while the leg is internally rotated. A radiograph should be obtained to check that the hip is concentrically reduced. Very rarely, open reduction is necessary (Pearson and Mann, 1973). After reduction, the leg should be immobilized in Russell traction with the hip in abduction. The duration of immobilization is debatable but several authors report that the hip was stable following reduction and that redislocation did not occur. Glass and Powell (1961) therefore suggested that it is harmless to bear weight 4 weeks after reduction. Early weight-bearing does not appear to influence the onset of complications.

Complications

Avascular necrosis is the most frequent. Glass and Powell (1961) noted that only 1 child out of 26 under the age of 10 years developed avascular change whereas 5 out of 20 children aged 10 years or more were affected. The incidence of avascular necrosis is about 10 per cent (Pennsylvania Orthopaedic Society, 1968). Rang (1974) stressed that prompt reduction will reduce the incidence of avascular necrosis and that this was only seen when reduction was delayed beyond 12 hours. The interval between injury and the diagnosis of this complication is seldom greater than one year (Haliburton, Brockenshire and Barber, 1961). Other rare problems mentioned in the literature are degenerative joint changes, premature epiphyseal fusion, overgrowth of the head of the femur (Glass and Powell, 1961) and sciatic nerve palsy (Pearson and Mann, 1973).

Results

About one-third of the hips showed some abnormality in the two series where results have been followed to maturity (Glass and Powell, 1961; Pennsylvania Orthopaedic Society, 1968). Simple dislocation of the hip in younger children almost always has a good result. A poor result is more likely in an adolescent child where the dislocation has been produced by severe trauma.

Acknowledgement

Fractures of the neck of the femur in children are very rare and few surgeons have had the opportunity of seeing more than three or four during their careers. The author is grateful to many sugeons who have referred patients or have allowed him to study the documents and radiographs of their cases. Without their kindness and help this work could not have been accomplished.

REFERENCES

Allende, G. and Lezama, L. G. (1951). Fractures of the neck of the femur in children – a clinical study. *J. Bone Jt Surg.* **33A**, 387

Barnes, R., Brown, J. T., Garden, R. S. and Nicholl, E.A. (1976). Subcapital fractures of the femur. *J. Bone Jt Surg.* **58B**, 2

Blount, W. P. (1955). *Fractures in Children*. Baltimore: The Williams and Wilkins Company; London: Bailliere, Tindall and Cox

Carrell, B. and Carrell, W. B. (1941). Fractures in the neck of the femur in children with particular reference to aseptic necrosis. *J. Bone Jt Surg.* **23**, 225

Catto, M. (1965). The histological appearances of late segmental collapse of the femoral head after transcervical fracture. *J. Bone Jt Surg.* **47B**, 777

Chong, K. C., Chacha, P. B. and Lee, B. T. (1976). Fractures of the neck of the femur in childhood and adolescence. *Injury* 111

Colonna, P. C. (1929). Fracture of the neck of the femur in children. *Am. J. Surg.* (N.S.) **6**, 793

Crenshaw, A. H. (1963). *Campbell's Operative Orthopaedics*. Vol. 1, p. 488. St. Louis: C.V. Mosby Co.

Durbin, F. C. (1959). Avascular necrosis complicating undisplaced fractures of the neck of the femur in children. *J. Bone Jt Surg.* **41B**, 758

Freeman, G. E. Jr (1961). Traumatic dislocation of the hip in children: a report of seven cases and review of the literature. *J. Bone Jt Surg.* **43A**: 401

Funk, F. J. Jr (1962). Traumatic dislocation of the hip in children. Factors influencing prognosis and treatment. *J. Bone Jt Surg.* **44A**, 1135

Glass, A. and Powell, H. D. W. (1961). Traumatic dislocation of the hip in children. An analysis of 47 patients. *J. Bone Jt Surg.* **43B**, 29

Green, J. T. (1960). Management of fresh fractures of the neck of the femur. *Instructional Course Lectures* **XVII**, p. 97. Saint Louis: C. V. Mosby Co.

Gupta, A. K. and Chaturvedi, S. N. (1973). *Indian J. Surg.* **35**, 567

Gupta, A. K., Chaturvedi, S. N. and Pruthi, K. K. (1975). Fracture of neck of femur in children. *Proc. Sicot* 4105

Haliburton, R. A., Brockenshire, F. A. and Barber, J. R. (1961). Avascular necrosis of the femoral capital epiphysis after traumatic dislocation of the hip in children. *J. Bone Jt Surg.* **43B**, 43

Harris, W. R. and Bobechko, W. P. (1960). The radiographic density of avascular bone. *J. Bone Jt Surg.* **42B**, 626

REFERENCES

Imhäuser, G. (1963). Der Schenkelhalsbruch des Kindes und seine Komplikationen – Insbesondere die Pseudarthrose. *Arch orthop Unfall Chir.* **55**, 274

Ingram, A. J. and Bachynski, B. (1953). Fractures of the hip in children. *J. Bone Jt Surg.* **35A**, 867

Kite, J. H., Lovell, W. W. and Allman, F. L. (1962). Fracture of the hip in the young. *J. Bone Jt Surg.* **44A**, 1710

Lam, S. F. (1964). Some aspects of fracture of the neck of the femur in children. *Singapore Med. J.* **5**, 179

Lam, S. F. (1965). Fractures of the neck of the femur in the young and their complications. *J. Western Pacific Orthop. Ass.* **II**, 1

Lam, S. F. (1971). Fractures of the neck of the femur in children. *J. Bone Jt Surg.* **53A**, ii, 1165

McDougall, A. (1961). Fractures of the neck of the femur in childhood. *J. Bone Jt Surg.* **43B**, 16

Mercer, W. and Duthie, R. B. (1964). *Orthopaedic Surgery* London: Edward Arnold

Meyers, M. H., Harvey, J. P. and Moore, T. M. (1973). Treatment of displaced subcapital and transcervical fractures of the femoral neck by muscle-pedicle bone-graft and internal fixation. *J. Bone Jt Surg.* **55A**, 257

Mitchell, J. I. (1936). Fracture of the neck of the femur in children. *J. Am. Med. Ass.* **107**, 1603

Morton, K. S. (1959). Traumatic dislocation of the hip. A follow-up study. *Can. J. Surg.* **3**, 67

Pearson, E. D. and Mann, R. J. (1973). Traumatic hip dislocation in children. *Clin. Orthopaed. Related Res.* **92**, 189

Peltokallio, P. and Kurkipää, M. (1959). Fractures of the femoral neck in children. *Ann. Chir. Gynaec. Fenniae* **48**, Suppl. 83–84, 151

Pennsylvania Orthopaedic Society (1968). Traumatic dislocation of the hip joint in children. *J. Bone Jt Surg.* **42A**, 705; **50A**, 79

Piggot, J. (1961). Traumatic dislocation of the hip in childhood. *J. Bone Jt Surg.* **43B**, 38

Rang, M. (1974). *Children's Fractures.* J. B. Lippincott Company

Ratliff, A. H. C. (1962). Avascular necrosis of the head of the femur after fractures of the femoral neck in children and Perthes' disease. *Proc. R. Soc. Med.* **55**, 504

Ratliff, A. H. C. (1962) Fractures of the neck of the femur in children. *J. Bone Jt Surg.* **44B**, 528

Ratliff, A. H. C. (1967). Fractures of the femoral neck in children. A clinical study of 120 cases. In *Dixieme Congres International de Chirurgie Orthopedique et de Traumatologie*, p. 151. Ed. M. J. Delchef. Bruxelles: Les publications 'Acta Medica Belgica'

Ratliff, A. H. C. (1968a). Fractures of the neck of the femur in children. A study of 132 cases. Ch.M. Thesis, University of Bristol

Ratliff, A, H. C. (1968b): Traumatic separation of the upper femoral epiphysis in young children. *J. Bone Jt Surg.* **50B**, 757

Rigault, P., Iselin, F., Moreau, J. and Judet, J. (1966). Fractures du col du femur chez l'Enfant. *Rev. Chir. orthop. reparatrice de l'Appareil Moteur* (Paris) **52**, 3, 325

Strange, F. G. St. C. (1965). *The Hip.* London: William Heinemann Medical Books Ltd

Talwalkar, C. A. (1974). Fracture of the femoral neck in children. Ch.M. Thesis, University of Liverpool

Trueta, J. (1957). The normal vascular anatomy of the human femoral head during growth. *J. Bone Jt Surg.* **39B**, 358

Watson-Jones, R. (1955). *Fractures and Joint Injuries.* Edinburgh and London: E. and S. Livingstone Ltd

Wilson, D. W. (1966). Traumatic dislocation of the hip in children: a report of four cases. *J. Trauma*, **6**, 739

199

6

Slipped Upper Femoral Epiphysis

A. H. C. Ratliff

The purpose of this chapter is to present the essential features of this condition with special reference to some of the aspects which are of topical debate at the present time. There is discussion on the aetiology, the direction and severity of the slipping, the interpretation of radiographs and the nature of the pre-slipping phase. While the clinical features are well described, nevertheless, the problem of how best to correct the severe slipped capital femoral epiphysis is as yet unsolved. The present diversity of treatment reflects dissatisfaction with the results obtained. There is always the fear of damage to the blood supply and more recently the subject of cartilage necrosis has received some attention. The literature on long-term follow-up of different methods requires discussion because it is still inadequate for accurate comparison of the results of different methods of treatment.

AETIOLOGY, PATHOLOGY AND NATURAL HISTORY

The condition of adolescent coxa vara or slipped upper femoral epiphysis usually occurs between the ages of 10 and 16 years (Burrows, 1957). There is a striking difference in age between the boys — mostly 14 to 16 years old — and the girls, mostly 11 to 13 years. It is more common in boys than girls (about 3 : 1). In Burrows' study (1957) none occurred under the age of 9 years. The upper limit of age-incidence coincides with the closure of the epiphyseal plate, but there are reports of patients with hormonal imbalance where displacement of the epiphysis occurred over the age of 20 years (Burrows, 1957; Simpson, 1950; Heatley, Greenwood, and Boase, 1976). There is bilateral involvement in 20 per cent. A girl who has started to menstruate is almost immune from slipping of the upper femoral epiphysis. In unilateral cases the condition is more common on the left side (Alexander, 1966). It is rare. The annual incidence of diagnosed cases among Connecticut residents was estimated to be 3.41 for 100 000 population under the age of 25 years (Kelsey, Keggi and Southwick, 1970).

Three typical types predominate: the adipose-genital; the long, thin rapidly growing boy; and a large group of children with an average physique for their sex and age. A precise distinction between those children with or without an endocrine defect is difficult and arbitrary. Burrows (1957) found 30 'constitutionally seemingly normal' out of a total of 73. Rather unexpectedly, no striking relationship was found between constitutional factors and bilateral affection.

A possible endocrine basis for slipping of the upper femoral epiphysis has been studied by Harris (1950) and supported by Lofgren (1953) and Theander (1962). Harris subjected the upper tibial epiphysis in the rat to shearing forces, which indicated the pressure at which they separated from the metaphysis. When the epiphysis separates from the diaphysis the plane of cleavage is constant, passing through the large cartilage cell layer of the epiphyseal plate. Sex hormones increased the shearing strength of the epiphyseal plate, whereas growth hormones decreased it. These changes were due to alteration produced by the two hormones in the thickness of the third layer of the plate. It was suggested that these findings may be of significance in providing an anatomical basis for slipping of the upper femoral epiphysis in man. In support of this suggestion is the fact that the problem only occurs in the weight-bearing epiphysis at the upper end of the femur subjected to shearing strain; it can be bilateral, and it may follow trivial injury. This is still a complicated subject since the precise action of other hormones such as testosterone on the epiphyseal plate is less clear. Further, it does not explain the normal state of other epiphyses (Burrows, 1957) and the existence of unilateral cases. This theory is supported by the report of a girl who, at the age of 15 years, had growth hormone deficiency — a slip of one femoral capital epiphysis developed at the age of 17 during growth-hormone therapy (Rennie and Mitchell, 1974). On the other hand, Razzona, Nelson and Eversman (1972) examined 5 patients with slipped femoral epiphysis (4 chronic, 1 acute) and found no abnormality of serum growth hormone or of 24-hour urinary oestrogen levels. This subject is made even more controversial by the recent paper of Heatley, Greenwood and Boase (1976). They describe 4 cases of slipped upper femoral epiphysis in patients with intracranial tumours causing hypopituitarism and chiasmal compression. Detailed endocrine studies in 3 cases showed severe deficiency of growth hormone as well as gonadotrophin and sex hormones. This hormonal background does not lend support to the hypothesis of Harris and they consider that there is no evidence that this mechanism operates in man.

In a further paper (Harris and Hobson, 1956), the histological changes in experimentally displaced upper femoral epiphyses in rabbits were studied. Through a posterior exposure the epiphysis was detached and then re-attached and held by a fine Kirschner wire introduced from the head into the neck. The animals were killed at weekly intervals up to 6 weeks and a comparison was made between the histological condition of the normal femoral head and that on which the operation was performed. It will be recalled that a normal epiphyseal plate consists of four distinct layers: resting cells, penetrating cells, hypertrophying cells and endochondral ossification. Harris and Hobson showed that there was a constant plane of cleavage and this plane was almost invariably through the area of hypertrophied cartilage on the diaphyseal side of the epiphyseal plate. Thus there now appears to be clear evidence on the histological site where displacement occurs. This displacement in some children may have an endocrine basis; in others, it may occur in constitutionally normal children subjected to an appreciable shearing strain. Ratliff (1968) described traumatic

201

separation of the upper femoral epiphysis in 13 apparently normal children all less than 9 years of age and subjected to severe violence (*see* Chapter 5).

There are other possible causes which have been suggested to explain the occurrence of slipped upper femoral epiphysis. Billing (1954) and Rennie (1960) suggested that deficient osteogenesis posteriorly produced obliquity of the cartilage plate. Rennie (1960) considered that the horizontal force generated by the standing posture caused the deficient osteogenesis, but Billing and Severin (1959) showed that the short posterior neck found in this condition was the result rather than the cause of the slipping.

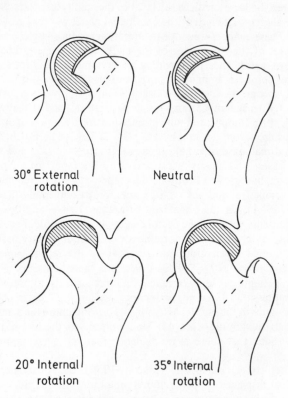

Figure 6.1. Diagram to illustrate the variable appearances which can result from an anteroposterior radiograph of a chronic slip in different positions of rotation
(Reproduced by permission from Griffith, 1976)

Alexander (1966) considered that the fundamental lesion of epiphysiolysis is a slow posterior migration of the head on the neck. Sitting shearing-stresses were measured and postulated as the likely cause of growth deviation. In the writing position, greater stress was taken on the left side in right-handed children. This theory is supported by the accepted fact that epiphysiolysis is commoner on the left side than the right (Key, 1926; Brailsford, 1953; Burrows, 1957; Howorth, 1957; and Theander, 1962). Though ingenious, it implies the unproved observation that most children sit more on the left side. Rennie (1967) noted a familial incidence of slipped upper femoral epiphysis and in the past 25 years there had been admitted to the Orthopaedic Service in Aberdeen 12 adolescents having a close relative who previously or subsequently developed slipped upper femoral epiphysis. He therefore believed that in this condition there is evidence of a genetic defect, probably due to a recessive gene of low penetrance. It has to be admitted that many theories have been suggested regarding the aetiology of slipped capital femoral epiphysis but the precise cause is not known.

There has been recent renewed interest on the subject of direction of displacement of the epiphysis. It is usually stated that the epiphysis is displaced postero-medially (Campbell, 1971) and indeed Murray and Duncan (1971) stated that pure posterior displacement only occurs in a few cases. On the other hand, Billing and Severin (1959) showed that in a series of 60 patients slipping occurred in a strictly posterior direction in relation to the neck. Griffith (1976) has recently re-examined this subject based on laboratory studies of the normal proximal ends of the femur of 6 children dying of unrelated disease and also of 45 patients with recent slipping of the upper femoral epiphysis. In the clinical studies, anteroposterior films were taken with the leg in varied directions of external and internal rotation. He stressed that variable appearances can result because of the anteversion plane of the neck of the femur (*Figure 6.1*).

Whenever a radiograph was taken with the leg internally rotated to the same degree as the anteversion plane of the neck of the femur, then the epiphysis lay directly behind the neck. On this evidence Griffith considers that the epiphyseal plate is an arc in the anteroposterior plane. The epiphysis is obliged to slip posteriorly by retreating along this arc of the growth plate and its assumed prolongation. There is no evidence that medial or lateral displacement occurs. Later, the anterior aspect of the neck becomes absorbed and new bone is laid down beneath the periosteum. Griffith (1976) believes that there is no true shortening of the posterior aspect of the neck and that so-called shortening is not due to deficient osteogenesis. If we accept these observations, they are an important advance for two reasons:

1. Radiographs must be taken in exactly the same way in order to compare the results of different methods of treatment. Griffith (1976) recommends that in both the anteroposterior and the lateral radiographs the x-ray should pass in the same plane as the epiphyseal plate. In order to obtain a true anteroposterior projection of the epiphyseal plate, the leg must be internally rotated by a degree equal to the amount of anteversion.

2. It is possible that the so-called triplane osteotomy for correction is not necessary.

When slipped upper femoral epiphysis occurs, the course is variable. Billing and Severin (1959) established that the head migrates posteriorly before radiographic evidence of frank slipping occurs. In this so-called pre-fracture stage without apparent displacement there is no loss of cartilage bone continuity and the only evidence is a plate-neck angle reduced below the normal of 90° (Howorth, 1949) (*Figure 6.2*).

In other cases, the femoral head moves backwards much more rapidly, exposing the anterior part of the end of the femoral neck (*Figure 6.6(a)*): the periosteum and vessels over the front of the neck are stretched. The epiphysis hinges on the posterior periosteum and the posterior border of the epiphysis may engage and eventually fuse with the superior quadrant of the neck. The vital epiphyseal blood vessels lie posteriorly and when damaged avascular necrosis may occur, though fortunately this is not common (*see later*). The stump of

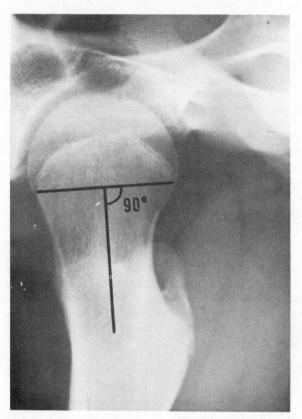

Figure 6.2. To illustrate the normal epiphyseal-plate angle (90°)

the neck is covered with calcified cartilage from the growth plate and epiphyseal fusion is usually premature. Heyman, Herndon and Strong (1957) stressed the production of new bone at the anterosuperior aspect of the neck of the femur at its junction with the displaced epiphysis and stated that this impinging on the edge of the acetabulum may restrict movement, particularly abduction and internal rotation (*Figure 6.7 (e)*). Herndon, Heyman and Bell (1963) stated that the average time required for fusion of the epiphyseal plate with conservative treatment is 19 months after the onset of symptoms.

CLINICAL FEATURES

Cardinal symptoms are pain and limp and these started simultaneously in half of those cases recorded by Burrows (1957). If either or both develop in adolescence in the years during which coxa vara occurs, then the diagnosis must be assumed. Pain usually presents in the region of the hip or the front of thigh. It is a common experience for pain to be referred to the knee though exactly why this should occur in this condition is not known. Pain is more often intermittent than continuous, dull and vague in character and exacerbated by sport. In about one-third of the cases there is a history of an injury. The common accident is a fall, often directly on to the affected hip, but sometimes a wrench. A careful history often elucidates mild and disregarded pain or limp followed by a fall with immediate disability. In these it is likely that sudden increased displacement has occurred.

The child may show one of the physical types already mentioned and, if so, a diagnosis is established. In some with mild pain and minimal disability, the only sign may be a terminal restriction of internal rotation. In others, often after a fall, the leg lies in fixed external rotation and slight adduction and walking may be impossible. These signs will clearly depend on the degree of displacement of the epiphysis. There may be shortening but seldom more than half an inch. Despite the well-known clinical features, delay in diagnosis and treatment often occurs. Newman (1960) stated that in his group of patients, all of whom were treated surgically, there was an average delay of 26 weeks from the initial onset of symptoms until the day of operation. Most of the delay occurred before the symptoms were reported to the patients' family doctor or school medical officer and the condition appeared trivial to the parents or had been dismissed as growing pains or rheumatism. In addition, there was delay in clinical diagnosis sometimes due to a false radiographic reassurance because of the lack of lateral views. Once the diagnosis had been made, there was still a delay of 3 to 8 weeks before an operation was performed. This subject has now become of medico-legal significance. I have recently been involved in the assessment of a legal claim where parents sued several general practitioners who failed to examine the hip of a child who had persistent pain in the knee for 6 months.

RADIOLOGICAL SIGNS

Radiological diagnosis is not easy in the early stage even with good radiographs and a normal opposite hip. Only widening of the epiphyseal line can be apparent in the anteroposterior view, described more precisely by Scott (1956) as juxta-epiphyseal osteoporosis in the metaphysis (*Figure 6.3 (a)*).

There is no convincing evidence that the osteoporosis precedes the slipping (Griffith, 1972). It is essential if there is doubt to take views in the lateral plane (*Figure 6.3 (b)*). The papers of Billing and Severin (1955, 1959) are notable contributions on this subject. A line drawn along the superior surface of the neck remains superior to the head instead of passing through it (Trethowan's sign). Griffith (1972) has recently stressed again that normally in the lateral view the epiphyseal plate and femoral neck lie at right-angles to each other — the lower limit of normal being $87°$ (*Figure 6.2*). When slipping is present the

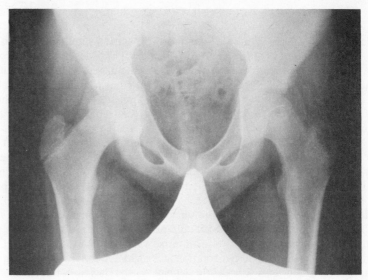

Figure 6.3. Boy aged 15. Early chronic slip less than one-third diamater of the neck treated by pinning with later bilateral involvement. (a) Note the porosis at the epiphyseal plate in the anteroposterior view left hip — easily missed. The right is normal

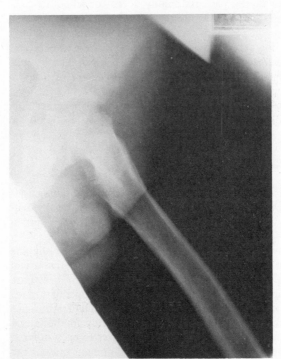

Figure 6.3. (b) Lateral view showing mild but definite posterior displacement

206

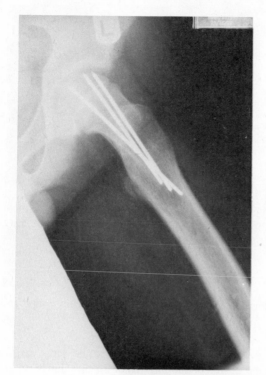

Figure 6.3. (c) Immediate pinning. The pins are marginally too long

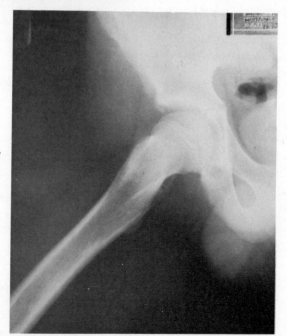

Figure 6.3. (d) Eleven months later. Pain in the right hip. Radiographs probably normal. Immediate pinning

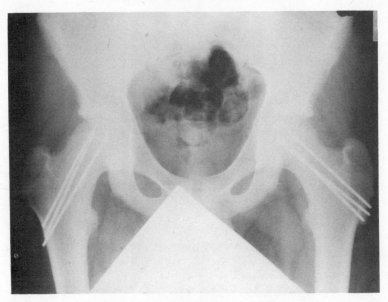

Figure 6.3. (e) Radiographs 3 years after first seen. An excellent clinical and radiological result. Note with growth the pins are not close to the joint

epiphyseal-plate angle becomes less than 87°. This is the most satisfactory method of determining the degree of slipping. Later, in this slowly progressive condition, adaptive changes take place in the neck of the femur. Bone is resorbed at the anterior margin of the neck and new bone formed on the posterior margin. Remodelling with growth may occur but, so far as I am aware, no detailed study of this fascinating subject has yet been made. The femoral head maintains its normal relationship with the acetabulum and in some severe cases the head may be displaced almost completely on to the posterior aspect of the neck.

TREATMENT

There now appears to be agreement on certain principles of management of this condition:

1. Whatever method of treatment is used, it is clear that the importance of an adequate blood supply to the upper femoral epiphysis must be kept constantly in mind; it is the most important factor in treatment (Newman, 1960) (*Figure 6.4*).
2. The disadvantages of conservative treatment which includes bed-rest and traction with internal rotation are numerous. It is doubted whether such treatment can reduce an epiphysis once it has become adherent, and further displacement can occur. In the series studied by Griffith (1972), further displacement developed in 25 per cent of those cases treated conservatively. Further, there is a prolonged morbidity with

disuse osteoporosis and a stiffened hip. This method is now generally considered to have no place in the treatment of this condition (Durbin, 1960; Newman, 1960).

3.   Because of the risk of further slipping, it seems rational now that the profession should regard slipped upper femoral epiphysis as a surgical emergency no matter what the degree of slip or the mildness of symptoms (Newman, 1960). Thus the main decision concerns the choice of operation only.

The prognosis for the type and degree of slip is very different and it is essential to have a simple classification (Newman, 1960). He divides cases into three groups.

Group 1.   Position of the epiphysis acceptable (65 per cent) (e.g. *Figure 6.3(a)*).

Group 2.   Position of the epiphysis unacceptable but epiphysis mobile (10 per cent) (*Figure 6.6 (a)*).

Group 3.   Position of epiphysis unacceptable and fixed (25 per cent).

It must be stressed that the majority of cases are in Group 1 and that their treatment is relatively easy. The epiphysis is stabilized *in situ* by the minor surgical procedure of internal fixation (*Figure 6.3*). An unacceptable degree of deformity has been defined as a displacement more than one-third the diameter of the neck in the lateral view (Wilson, 1938) (e.g. *Figure 6.6 (a)*). However, the author has seen cases where even greater displacement has been fixed *in situ* and then, apparently, remodelling has occurred with growth to produce quite satisfactory results (*Figure 6.5 (a)*). A large nail should never be used since forcible hammering may be necessary, leading to further displacement of the epiphysis and predisposing to subtrochanteric fracture. Fixation should be by two or three pins of the Newman or Smith-Petersen guide-wire variety. Moore's pins are now no longer popular because of the occasional difficulty in later removal after new bone formation around the pin. The pins recommended are easily inserted, especially when controlled on a powered electric drill with minimal trauma, and can cross the posterior cortex of the neck of the femur if necessary (*Figure 6.5 (a)*). Weight-bearing may be permitted after three weeks. The prognosis for the chronic slip with mild displacement that can be fixed *in situ* is usually good though very occasionally avascular necrosis may occur (Hall, 1957). In all the remaining patients, i.e. approximately one-third of the total (Newman, 1960), the position of the epiphysis was unacceptable. In these cases it has to be ascertained whether the epiphysis is mobile so that the position can be improved. There is always anxiety concerning possible damage of the blood supply of the epiphysis which lies within the synovial reflection on the posterior aspect of the neck. Changes may then involve the whole or segments of the epiphysis resulting in avascular necrosis, and the result of treatment is then almost always poor. Damage may, alternatively, occur to the articular cartilage alone, resulting in the condition of chondrolysis and a stiff, often deformed, painful hip.

The value of manipulation

In the acute traumatic slip, and the acute on chronic slip, the head is loose; providing no more than 3 weeks have elapsed since the acute episode, a gentle manipulation of the flexed hip in internal rotation can produce an improvement in the anatomical position (Fahey and O'Brien, 1965). Griffith (1972) considered that the proportion of successful reductions has been overestimated by some authors since they have had variable views when studying the radiographs. In his series (1976) the position was improved in 38 per cent, but avascular necrosis ensued in 73 per cent of those successfully manipulated. Avascular necrosis did not occur in any of the hips manipulated without any improvement in the position of the epiphysis. Dunn (1975), with an exceptional experience of this subject, believes there is no such thing as a gentle manipulation of the retinacular vessels.

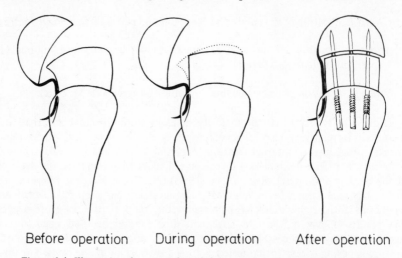

Before operation   During operation   After operation

Figure 6.4. Illustrating the principles of the operation advocated by Dunn. Note the exposed anterior part of the neck, the posterior position of the epiphyseal blood vessels and the shortened neck

On the other hand, a recent meeting of the British Orthopaedic Association (Griffith, 1975) revealed that this was still a very controversial subject and some authors have suggested that this procedure is still of value (Newman, 1960; Vaughan-Jackson, 1965; Fairbank, 1969). All seem agreed that the manipulation should be gentle, and should never be attempted on the chronic severe slip without an acute episode. After replacement, internal fixation should be performed under the same anaesthetic providing the position achieved is acceptable.

If manipulation fails or the position of the epiphysis is unacceptable and fixed, then the essential alternatives are to perform an osteotomy of the femoral neck, a subtrochanteric or intertrochanteric osteotomy, or to fuse the epiphysis and remove the exostosis.

In cervical osteotomy the basic aim is removal of a wedge of bone based anteriorly from the femoral neck in order to bring the head into better relationship. Variations in technique include cuneiform or trapezoidal osteotomies, division of the femoral neck both proximal and distal, and followed by plaster casts or internal fixation. Griffith (1972) carried out a comprehensive review of the literature and studied the reported results of 19 separate papers. Out of 444 cervical osteotomies no fewer than 145 (33 per cent) had unsatisfactory results, most being due to avascular or cartilage necrosis. The indications for this operation are rare; it is not easy, and in general it is not often advised at the present time. Dunn (1964), however, points out, 'whereas the intertrochanteric operation leaves the anatomy of the hip grossly abnormal, cervical osteotomy makes it nearly normal again'. He considered that the late onset of degenerative arthritis was more likely after the former operation. In 1964, Dunn introduced a modified open reduction and cervical osteotomy. In this operation, the great trochanter is detached, the retinacular vessels are carefully mobilized by gentle subperiostial dissection, the neck is shortened, and the epiphysis fixed by pins (*Figure 6.4*).

Dunn has had a unique experience and has stressed when not to do the operation, i.e. in the case of a severe chronic slip with the growth plate closed. He points out that one of the most difficult decisions is to decide if the plate is still open or not. The result of 73 open replacement operations followed-up for an average of 7 years has been recently described (Dunn, 1975). Avascular necrosis, complete or segmental, occurred in 14 per cent. Narrowing of the joint space suggestive of chondrolysis occurred in 18 per cent. Thus, it may be concluded that this operation is not an easy one, even for the expert,

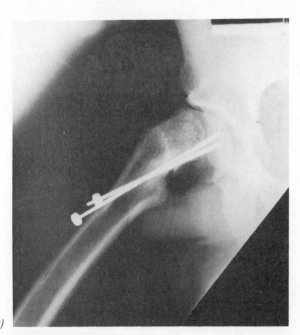

(a)

Figure 6.5. Acute on chronic slip treated by pinning. To illustrate the result of treatment with an 11 year follow-up of a boy aged 14 at the time of injury. Gentle manipulation and internal fixation. No endocrine defect. (a) Radiograph 4 months after internal fixation

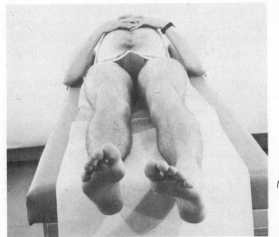

(b)

(c)

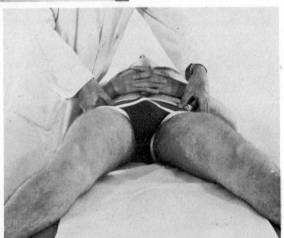

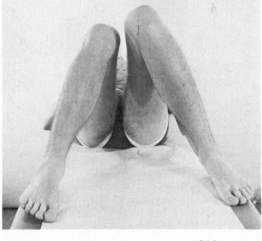

(d)

Figure 6.5. (b) (c) (d) He is now 6ft 1in, aged 25, no complaints, delighted. Works as an insurance inspector. Flexion full. Clinically there is some blemish, notably 1 inch of shortening, slight restriction of abduction

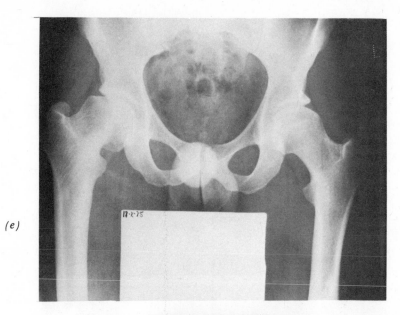

(e)

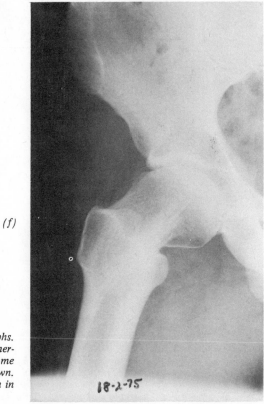

(f)

Figure 6.5. (e) (f) Recent radiographs. Will this young man develop degenerative arthritis in the years to come and if so when? Answer unknown. (Further pictures have been taken in 1976 and show no change)

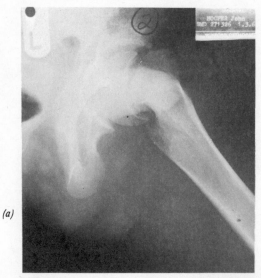

(a)

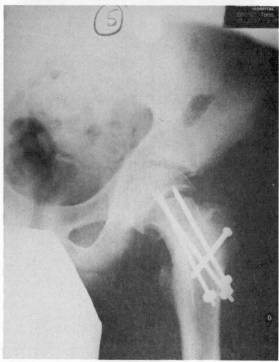

(b)

Figure 6.6. An acute slip with gross displacement treated by Dunn osteotomy and pinning. The result of treatment with a 9-year follow-up of a boy aged 16 at the time of injury. Some evidence of delayed hormonal development. (a) An acute slip with gross unacceptable displacement. (b) Radiographs immediately after operation

214

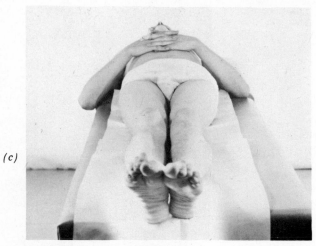

(c)

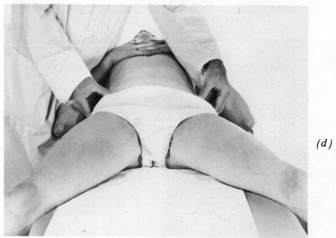

(d)

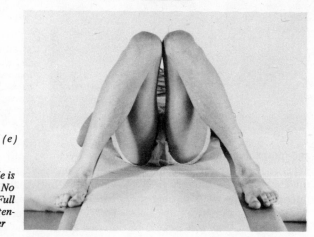

(e)

Figure 6.6. (c) (d) (e) He is now 5ft 9in, aged 26. No clinical abnormality. Full movements and no shortening. Works as a butcher

215

(f)

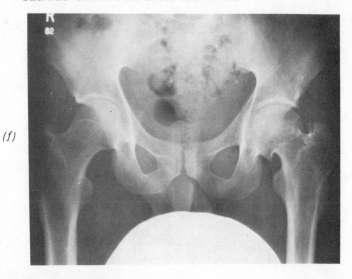

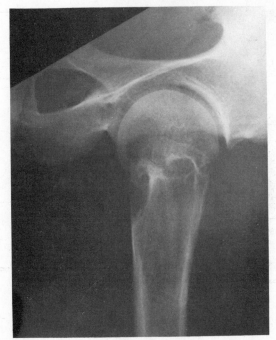

(g)

Figure 6.6. (f) (g) Minor lipping and a 'coarse' appearance of the head with a slightly short neck. Will this young man develop degenerative arthritis in the years to come and if so when? Answer unknown

and probably should not be done except by those with special and frequent experience. Providing avascular necrosis does not develop, the author has noted the apparently satisfactory results without deformity that may be obtained with internal fixation of a chronic slip where the displacement is greater than one-third of the diameter of the neck. Two similar cases are illustrated in *Figures 6.5*, and *6.6*. One was treated by internal fixation and the other by cervical osteotomy and internal fixation. Both are very good clinically as far as the patient is concerned ten years later, though the patient with a cervical osteotomy has a greater range of movements. The reader is left to make up his own mind on the advantages and disadvantages of each operation. I believe that a careful study of remodelling with growth over the years and strictly comparable radiographs, as described by Griffith, is necessary before this debate can be resolved.

Heyman, Herndon and Strong (1957) described a comparatively simple and conservative operation to remove the bony obstruction on the front of the neck of the femur. This is a useful measure in patients with a severe chronic slip and simply aims to improve movement. Later, Herndon, Heyman and Bell (1963) described the use of a bone graft across the epiphyseal plate as well as removal of the bony prominence. The aim was to produce an epiphyseodesis and reduce the immobilization to 12 weeks but to accept the deformity. The long-term results are not known.

If the epiphyseal plate is closed and the deformity appreciable it is now agreed that cervical osteotomy is dangerous and the alternatives are intertrochanteric or subtrochanteric osteotomy. The deformity is corrected by abduction and internal rotation at the osteotomy site. The results of trochanteric osteotomy are, on the whole, disappointing though the advantage is that the functional result may be satisfactory and there is no further risk of avascular necrosis or chondrolysis. Out of a total of 200 cases, 28 per cent were unsatisfactory (Griffith, 1972). Pearson and Riddell (1964) reviewed the results of 25 subtrochanteric osteotomies and stated that osteoarthritis tended to occur 8 to 15 years after this operation. Newman (1960) introduced the conception of triplane osteotomy with a flexion component to correct hyperextension as well as correction of the other two deformities. The results have recently been reported (Ireland and Newman, 1976). They reviewed the results of 34 operations observed for an average of 7 years. There were 28 good clinical results but nearly half of the good hips had an incomplete correction of the deformity. Poor results followed chondrolysis but there was no case of femoral-head necrosis. Southwick (1967) reported the technique of a biplane osteotomy at the level of the lesser trochanter. He deliberately corrected the deformity by producing a reversed deformity at a lower level. A lateral- and also anterior-based wedge is used to correct alignment. Thus, it is clear that the problem of how best to correct the severe, slipped capital femoral epiphysis is as yet unsolved. There are no adequately documented series of cases followed for 30 to 40 years and this is essential to judge what treatment gives the best results in this controversial subject.

COMPLICATIONS

Avascular necrosis

This complication influences the end result more than any other single factor. It occurred in 15 per cent of those described by Hall (1957). A poor result is not inevitable after loss of epiphyseal blood supply but it is usual. The author is not aware of any recent advances in the management of avascular necrosis complicating slipped upper femoral epiphysis. Total or segmental necrosis may occur. Like avascular necrosis after a fracture of the neck of the femur in children, it may be associated with a reasonably-functioning hip for some years. A subtrochanteric osteotomy may possibly be of benefit with relief of symptoms (*Figure 6.7 (f)*) so that further surgical procedures such as arthrodesis may be postponed indefinitely or at least until early adult life. Later, however, when symptoms become disabling, arthrodesis of the hip is the single most effective operative procedure for permanent relief of pain and satisfactory function especially in the young male with unilateral disease.

Chondrolysis

The condition of cartilage necrosis is now a recognized important complication of slipped upper femoral epiphysis. It was originally described by Waldenstrom (1930). He considered the pathology to be a disturbance of the function of the synovial lining in the joint with resultant death of the cartilage. This is supported

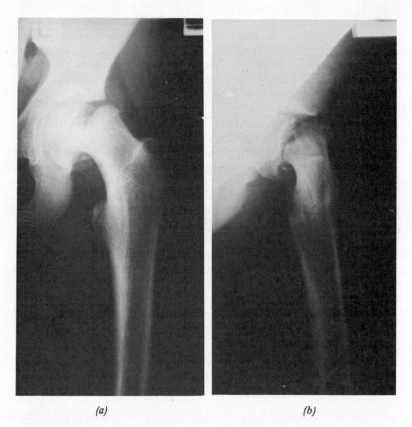

(a)   (b)

Figure 6.7. To illustrate avascular necrosis and one possible method of treatment. A girl aged 12 with a 5-month history of pain and an acute on chronic slip. No endocrine abnormality. (a) Anteroposterior radiograph. The slip is apparently posterior and medially. (b) The lateral view showing that the slip is posterior

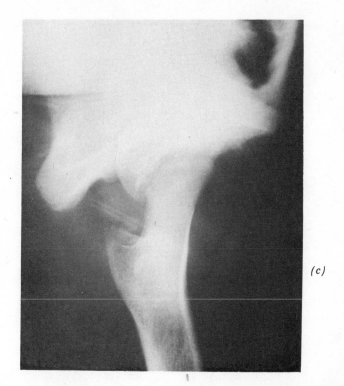

(c)

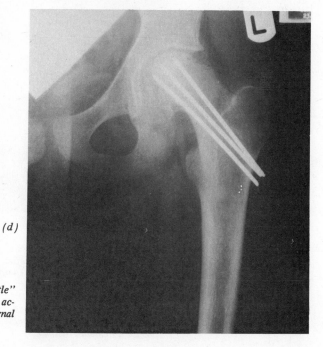

(d)

Figure 6.7. (c) "Gentle" manipulation position acceptable. (d) After internal fixation

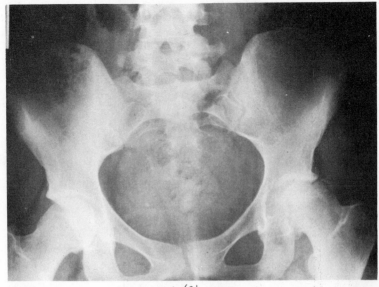

(e)

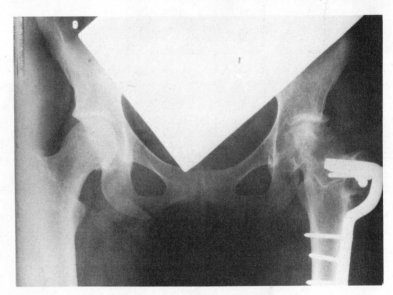

(f)

Figure 6.7. (e) Avascular necrosis developed 9 months after operation and this view was taken 5 years after initial treatment. Note the characteristic new bone on the superior aspect of the neck. Treatment necessary for pain and loss of movement. (f) One year after a subtrochanteric valgus osteotomy. This girl was delighted with the reduction of pain though there is still restriction of movement. Will arthrodesis eventually be necessary? Answer, probably yes, but no more precise statement possible

by Cruess (1963) who examined the pathology in two cases. Some studies suggested that race may play a part since the condition particularly occurs in negroes (Cruess, 1963; Orofino, Innis and Lowrey, 1960; and Golding, 1973). The reported occurrences of cartilage necrosis in other countries with a small negro population suggest that this may not be an important factor (Jerre, 1950; Hall, 1957; Durbin, 1960; and Lowe, 1961). The condition is usually rare but Golding (1973) described an incidence of 19 out of 47 hips, the majority affecting females, all presenting with pain and stiffness of insidious onset apparently unassociated with trauma. The condition progressed to produce a flexion deformity of the hip, sometimes with an abduction or an adduction contracture. The radiographic features were osteoporosis, joint-space narrowing, and erosion of the fovea. Early closure of the growth plate, often with some enlargement of the femoral head and neck was characteristic. Investigations had excluded tuberculosis and rheumatoid arthritis. The blood sedimentation rate, latex fixation test and blood count were normal except for the frequent appearance of an eosinophilia. Lowe (1970) stated that this complication usually arises within the first year after the diagnosis of slipping — sometimes within a few weeks. It can arise spontaneously after a slipping of the femoral epiphysis without any treatment and may follow slight or severe slip. There is no sex distinction and puberty proceeds normally.

The treatment is debatable. The prognosis after chondrolysis has been thought to be poor and arthrodesis, arthroplasty or osteotomy have often been carried out. Lowe (1970) described 6 cases where there was gradual return of joint space and considered the prognosis is therefore not always as bad as supposed. Golding (1973) also advised caution with regard to surgical treatment as most cases appear to recover spontaneously. An example of this condition is shown in *Figure 6.8*.

The treatment of the opposite hip

It is well recognized that during the treatment of a slipped upper femoral epiphysis the opposite hip may develop the same condition (*Figure 6.3 (d)*). Nearly a quarter of the cases are bilateral or become so after 6 to 24 months or more (Jerre, 1950; Burrows, 1957). In bilateral hips the average duration of symptoms for the first side was 26 weeks, while that for the second hip was 6 weeks (Hayes and Spitzer, 1975). Thus prophylactic pinning of the uninvolved hip of patients with an already-slipped epiphysis warrants consideration particularly when the involved epiphysis has slipped significantly and requires a major surgical procedure. This subject is controversial; some believe that it is justified to subject the patient to a relatively safe procedure on his normal hip, others that it is unnecessary. Most orthopaedic surgeons will agree that awareness of the possibility must be kept constantly in mind and that patients must be warned to return immediately if any symptoms develop, however mild, in the opposite hip. If there are symptoms, and particularly if the epiphyseal plate is widened and irregular, then pinning should be performed as a relative emergency.

The relation of bilateral affection to endocrine abnormality appears to have received little attention. Burrows (1957) stated that bilateral affection was no commoner in the endocrine group. O'Driscoll (1976) has investigated 37 cases of

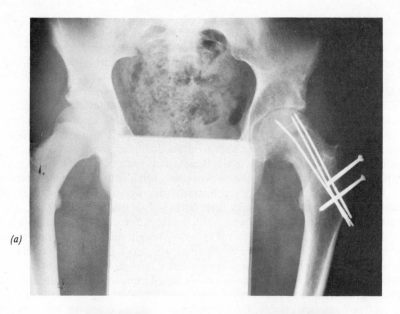

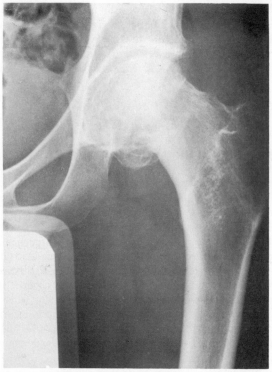

*Figure 6.8. An example of chondrolysis. (a) Radiograph
3 months after operation in a boy aged 14. (b) The same
hip 2½ years later, with some avascular necrosis*

slipped upper femoral epiphysis by studying their bone age and urinary-steroid and ketogenic-steroid excretion. In 26 unilateral cases with normal bone age and urinary steroids, the epiphyseal plate closed after pinning within 6 months and there was no contralateral slip. In 5 unilateral cases with both immature bone age and abnormal urinary steroids, a contralateral slip occurred within 1 year. There were 3 patients with gross hormonal abnormality (1 with hypopituitarism, 2 with hypogonadism) and of these the condition was bilateral in 2, unilateral in 1. There were 3 bilateral cases at presentation, and of these 2 were skeletally immature. O'Driscoll concluded that unilateral cases which were mature did not develop a contralateral slip. Prophylactic contralateral pinning was only indicated in those patients who were immature. These observations are interesting and helpful but full assessment of the clinical, radiological and endocrine condition of the patient is essential before this difficult decision is made. In all cases where the slip is bilateral with deficiencies of growth and sex hormones it is emphasized that surgical treatment can provide only temporary fixation because fusion is dependent on correct hormonal therapy. Treatment is complex and multi-disciplinary. In my opinion, expert medical advice is essential.

RESULTS OF TREATMENT

The short-term results of treatment were discussed by Hall (1957). He reviewed 173 hips observed for 5 years. 23 per cent were classified as fair or poor, avascular necrosis being the commonest cause of a poor result. This complication developed in 37 per cent of cases in which a manipulation was followed by a nailing operation, and for 38 per cent of cases of cervical osteotomy. Thus the results of treatment, even in those observed for a short period, are not encouraging and much still needs to be learned on this subject.

It is perhaps surprising that no long-term results are known and hence the incidence of degenerative arthritis is unknown. Jerre (1950) provided some useful information when he studied 183 hips observed for an average of 15 years. The functional results were classified as fair (39 per cent) and poor (23 per cent). As would be expected, the extent of epiphyseal displacement during adolescence had a pronounced influence on the late functional result and this became worse with increasing age. Finally, Jerre (1950) discussed the late radiological results. 'Arthrosis deformans' was very common among those cases with no symptoms at all (e.g. *Figure 6.5 (e)* and *(f)*). Pronounced symptoms were not seen without co-existent deformity of the hip. Deformation was observed in 75 per cent of the hips. No clear comparison can be made between this work and the recorded late results of Perthes' disease; a general impression is, however, obtained from this study, namely that the results are worse than those of Perthes' disease. Possibly this is due to the condition occurring in an older age group, which had less chance of remodelling with growth.

In preparing this chapter, the author has been surprised to note, on the one hand, the very large bibliography of this condition and yet, on the other, how much is still not known about the condition of slipped upper femoral epiphysis in the child.

Acknowledgement

The author is grateful to colleagues in Bristol for allowing him to study their cases of slipped upper femoral epiphysis and for their helpful comments.

REFERENCES

Alexander, C. (1966). The etiology of femoral epiphysial slipping. *J. Bone Jt Surg.* **48B,** 229

Billing, L. (1955). Roentgen examination of the proximal femur end in children and adolescents. *Acta radiol.* **Suppl. 110**

Billing, L. and Severin, E. (1959). Slipping epiphysis of the hip. *Acta radiol.* **Suppl. 174**

Brailsford, J. F. (1953). *The Radiology of Bones and Joints.* Fifth edn. London: J. & A. Churchill Ltd

Burrows, H. J. (1957). Slipped upper femoral epiphysis. *J. Bone Jt Surg.* **39B,** 641

Campbell's Operative Orthopaedics (1971), 5th Edn. St. Louis: C. V. Mosby Company p. 1061

Cruess, R. L. (1963). The pathology of acute necrosis of cartilage in slipping of the capital femoral epiphysis. *J. Bone Jt Surg.* **45A,** 1013

Dunn, Denis M. (1964). The treatment of adolescent slipping of the upper femoral epiphysis. *J. Bone Jt Surg.* **46B,** 621

Dunn, D. M. (1975). Severe slipped capital femoral epiphysis and open replacement by cervical osteotomy. *Proc. 3rd Open Scientific Meeting Hip Soc. St. Louis,* p. 115

Durbin, F. C. (1960). Treatment of slipped upper femoral epiphysis. *J. Bone Jt Surg.* **42B,** 289

Fahey, J. F. and O'Brien, E. T. (1965). Acute slipped capital femoral epiphysis: review of the literature and report of 10 cases. *J. Bone Jt Surg.* **47A,** 1105

Fairbank, T. J. (1969). Manipulative reduction of slipped upper femoral epiphysis. *J. Bone Jt Surg.* **51B,** 252

Golding, J. S. R. (1973). Chondrolysis of the hip. *J. Bone Jt Surg.* **55B,** 214

Griffith, M. J. (1972). Anatomical considerations in the treatment of slipping of the capital femoral epiphysis. M.Ch. Thesis, University of Liverpool.

Griffith, M. J. (1975). The morphology of slipped upper femoral epiphysis. *J. Bone Jt Surg.* **55B,** 653

Griffith, M. J. (1976). Slipping of the capital femoral epiphysis. *Ann. R. Coll. Surg.* **58,** 34

Hall, J. E. (1957). The results of treatment of slipped femoral epiphysis. *J. Bone Jt Surg.* **39B,** 659

Harris, W. R. (1950). The endocrine basis for slipping of the upper femoral epiphysis. An experimental study. *J. Bone Jt Surg.* **32B,** 5

Harris, W. R. and Hobson, K. W. (1956). Histological changes in experimentally displaced upper femoral epiphyses in rabbits. *J. Bone Jt Surg.* **38B,** 914

Hayes, M. G. and Spitzer, A. G. (1975). Slipped upper femoral epiphysis – a ten-year review. *J. Bone Jt Surg.* **57B,** 117

Heatley, F. W., Greenwood, R. H. and Boase, D. L. (1976). Slipping of the upper femoral epiphyses in patients with intracranial tumours causing hypopituitarism and chiasmal compression. *J. Bone Jt Surg.* **58B,** 169

Herndon, C. H., Heyman, C. H. and Bell, D. M. (1963). Treatment of slipped capital femoral epiphysis by epiphyseodesis and osteoplasty of the femoral neck. A report of further experiences. *J. Bone Jt Surg.* **45A,** 999

Heyman, C. H., Herndon, C. H. and Strong, J. M. (1957). Slipped femoral epiphysis with severe displacement. *J. Bone Jt Surg.* **39,** 298

Howorth, M. B. (1949). Slipping of the upper femoral epiphysis. *J. Bone Jt Surg.* **31A,** 734

Howorth, M. B. (1957). Slipping of the upper femoral epiphysis. *Clin. Orthop.* **10,** 148

Ireland, J. and Newman, P. H. (1976). Triplane osteotomy for severely slipped upper femoral epiphysis. *Proc. Sixth Combined Meeting Orthop. Ass. English-Speaking World*

Jerre, Torsten (1950). A study in slipped upper femoral epiphysis with special reference to the late functional and roentgenological results and to the value of closed reduction. *Acta. Orthop. Scand.* **Suppl. 6**

Kelsey, J. L., Keggi, K. J. and Southwick, W. O. (1970). The incidence of distribution of slipped capital femoral epiphysis in Connecticut and South Western United States, *J. Bone Jt Surg.* **52A,** 1203

REFERENCES

Key, T. A. (1926). Epiphysial coxa vara or displacement of the capital epiphysis of the femur of adolescence. *J. Bone Jt Surg.* **8**, 53

Lofgren, L. (1953). Slipping of the upper femoral epiphysis, signs of endocrine disturbance, size of sella turcica, and two illustrative cases of simultaneous slipping of the upper femoral epiphysis and tumour of the hypophysis. *Acta. Chir. Scand.* **106**, 153

Lowe, H. G. (1961). Avascular necrosis after slipping of the upper femoral epiphysis. *J. Bone Jt Surg.* **43B**, 688

Lowe, H. G. (1970). Necrosis of articular cartilage after slipping of the capital femoral epiphysis. Report of 6 cases with recovery. *J. Bone Jt Surg.* **52B**, 108

Murray, R. O. and Duncan, C. (1971). Athletic activity in adolescence as an etiological factor in degenerative hip disease. *J. Bone Jt Surg.* **53B**, 406

Newman, P. H. (1960). The surgical treatment of slipping of the upper femoral epiphysis. *J. Bone Jt Surg.* **42B**, 280

O'Driscoll, M. J. (1976). Personal communications

Orofino, C., Innis, J. J. and Lowrey, C. W. (1960). Slipped femoral epiphysis in Negroes. A study of 95 cases. *J. Bone Jt Surg.* **42A**, 1079

Pearson, J. R. and Riddell, D. M. (1964). Subtrochanteric osteotomy in the treatment of slipped upper femoral epiphysis. *J. Bone Jt Surg.* **42B**, 155

Ratliff, A. H. C. (1968). Traumatic separation of the upper femoral epiphysis in young children. *J. Bone Jt Surg.* **50B**, 757

Razzona, C. D., Nelson, C. and Eversman, J. (1972). *J. Bone Jt Surg.* **54A**, ii, 1224

Rennie, A. M. (1960). The pathology of slipped upper femoral epiphysis: a new concept. *J. Bone Jt Surg.* **42B**, 273

Rennie, A. M. (1967). Familial slipped upper femoral epiphysis. *J. Bone Jt Surg.* **49B**, 535

Rennie, W. and Mitchell, N. (1974). Slipped femoral capital epiphysis occurring during growth hormone therapy. *J. Bone Jt Surg.* **56B**, 703

Scott, J. C. (1956). *Displacement of the Upper Epiphysis of the Femur. Mod. Trends Orthop.*, Second Series p. 246. London: Butterworth

Simpson, S. L. (1950). Endocrinology and orthopaedics in fifty years. *J. Bone Jt Surg.* **32B**, 730

Southwick, W. C. (1967). Osteotomy through the lesser trochanter for slipped capital femoral epiphysis. *J. Bone Jt Surg.* **49A**, 807

Theander, G. (1962). Pelvic instability in upper femoral epiphysiolysis. *Acta Orthop. Scand.* **32**, 52

Vaughan-Jackson, O. J. (1965). Reducibility of slipped capital femoral epiphysis. *Proc. R. Soc. Med.* (Section of Orthopaedics) **49**, 812

Waldenstrom, H. (1930). On necrosis of the joint cartilage by epiphysiolysis capitis femoris. *Acta Chir. Scand.* **67**, 936

Wilson, P. D. (1938). The treatment of slipping of the upper femoral epiphysis with minimal displacement. *J. Bone Jt Surg.* **20**, 379

7

Miscellaneous

A. THE SIGNIFICANCE OF GENERALIZED DISORDERS OF THE SKELETON AS MIRRORED IN THE HIP

General disorders of the skeleton commonly involve the hip joint and merit attention for three reasons: firstly, for recognition that the malformation is part of a generalized disorder rather than one confined to the hip; secondly, because some require treatment in their own right; lastly, they are, by definition, generalized and we must remember the possibility of the presence or the development of some serious associated condition.

It may therefore be useful to classify these anomalies as to the manner in which they present in the context of the hip joint to the orthopaedic surgeon, mentioning briefly indications for treatment and important complicating features occurring elsewhere in the body. It is neither necessary nor desirable to memorize the general characteristics of these disorders which are becoming increasingly difficult to retain as new syndromes are recognized and old ones reclassified. There are good accounts in standard reference books of which those of Rubin (1964), Spranger, Langer and Wiedemann (1974), and Wynne-Davies and Fairbank (1976), will be found particularly helpful. They also provide selected references for further reading.

1. Delay in ossification of the capital epiphysis.

Delay in the appearance of the ossific nucleus will cause concern at six months and at one year indicates that an abnormality is present. Some delay is a feature of many general disorders but some are of special significance.

Cretinism is rightly well recognized as a cause, for replacement therapy is urgently required. Suspicion is reinforced by the characteristic facies and the wedge-shaped lower thoracic or upper lumbar vertebrae (*Figure 7.1*). The *Mucopolysaccharidoses*, especially the Morquio and Hurler varieties, may show prolonged delay and, indeed, provide the clue to diagnosis when more general features are tardy in appearing. Mental deterioration and early death are probable in Hurler's disease, whereas some patients with Morquio's syndrome live for many years and we must be aware of the risk of atlanto-axial dislocation due to odontoid hypoplasia. In *Stippled epiphyses* (Chondrodysplasia punctata) the

A. THE SIGNIFICANCE OF GENERALIZED DISORDERS

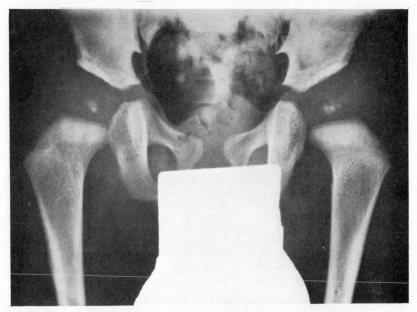

Figure 7.1. Cretin to show epiphyseal delay at 2 years and 3 months

characteristic stippling may not appear for two to three years and although usually confined to the epiphyses it may spread outwards into soft tissue, thereby explaining the contractures. Scoliosis, congenital cataract, and mental retardation are features of those who survive. *Dysplasia multiplex epiphysealis* is more commonly seen than those mentioned above. Delay is followed by irregular fragmented development and finally deformity of the epiphyses.

2. Coxa vara

Coxa vara may develop spontaneously, as a result of bone softening or following a fracture. In *Craniocleidodysostosis* developmental coxa vara is seen in association with a defect at the pubic symphysis *(Figure 7.2)*. Rarely, coxa vara may be caused by a congenital pseudarthrosis at subtrochanteric level. Softening which affects stability so that coxa vara develops under the pressure of body weight is seen in *Nutritional rickets* and more importantly in *Hypophosphataemic (Vitamin-D resistant) rickets (see Figures 7.30, 7.31)*. In the latter the prognosis for both growth and progressive deformity is directly related to the age at which the diagnosis is made and high doses of Vitamin D are prescribed. Distinction from *Metaphyseal dysostosis* may not be possible from radiographs alone but the level of the serum phosphate will decide *(Figure 7.3)*. *Hypophosphatasia* with a congenital lack of alkaline phosphatase may simulate severe rickets. If Craniostenosis is unrelieved it may lead to blindness in those that survive. The mother's phosphatase levels should be assessed in the interest of genetic counselling. *Hyperphosphatasia* is the synonym for juvenile Paget's disease and exhibits high levels of alkaline phosphatase. Deformities are similar to those seen in the

227

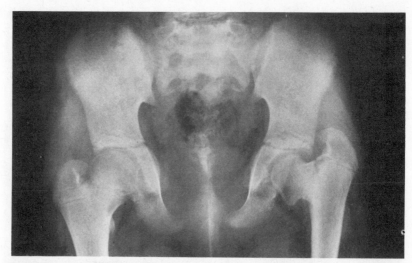

Figure 7.2. Craniocleidodysostosis. (a) There is coxa vara and on the left a pseudarthrosis of the femoral neck. Note the defective pubic symphysis

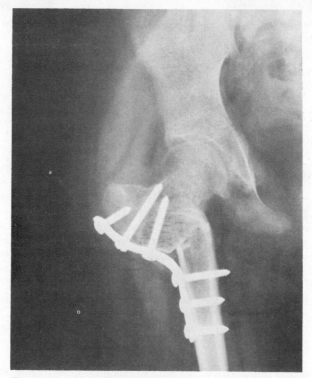

Figure 7.2. (b) Following corrective osteotomy at 11 years the pseudarthrosis is healed. The upper screw has been deliberately placed through the trochanteric epiphyseal plate to reduce the risk of recurrence

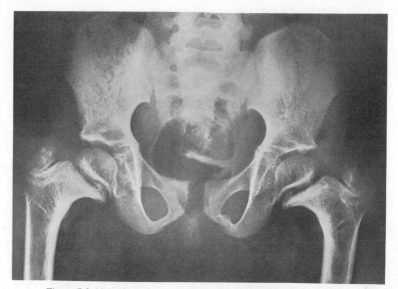

Figure 7.3. Metaphyseal dysostosis. Note the resemblance to rickets

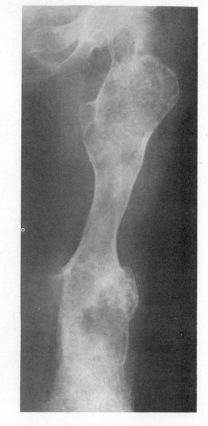

Figure 7.4. Dyschondroplasia. Note deformity of femoral head and cartilaginous masses in the femur. There is coxa valga

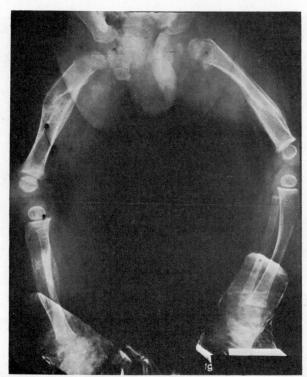

Figure 7.5. Osteogenesis imperfecta. (a) Multiple fractures; note the trochanteric fractures on the left

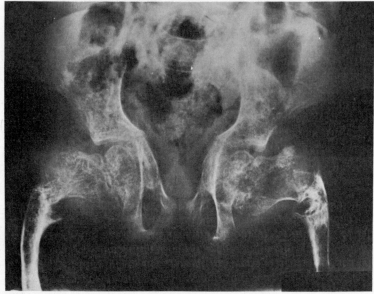

Figure 7.5. (b) Ten years later there is bilateral coxa vara and deformity of the pelvis

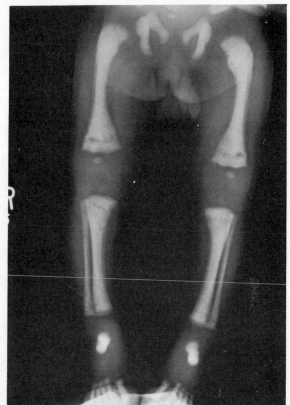

Figure 7.6. Osteopetrosis. At 4 months trochanteric fractures are visible in the abnormally dense bone. Note the characteristic translucent line in the metaphysis

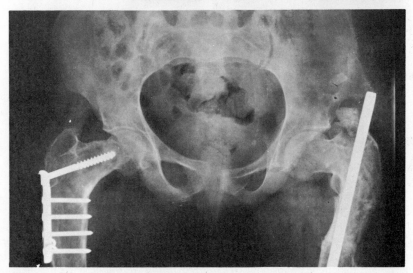

Figure 7.7. Fibrous dysplasia. Internal fixation has been used on the right to stabilize a trochanteric crack fracture. Coxa vara has developed on the left secondary to a sub-trochanteric fracture in spite of nailing

adult form and characteristic transverse fractures may contribute to them. These children are short-lived, gravely handicapped and develop leontiasis ossea with cranial nerve involvement. *Ollier's disease* (dyschondroplasia), if involving the proximal femur, may cause coxa vara due to the yielding of unossified cartilage. Fractures may contribute. The pituitary fossa may be involved affecting the function of the gland (*Figure 7.4*).

Coxa vara following fractures through abnormal bone is common, for the subtrochanteric level is often involved and, once deformity has occurred, mechanical factors encourage recurrence. This is frequently seen in *Osteogenesis imperfecta* and is a frequent indication for intramedullary nailing (*Figure 7.5*).

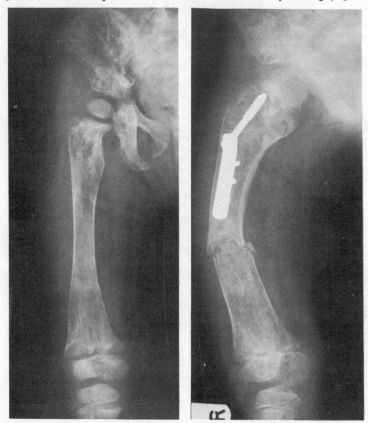

Figure 7.8. Albright's syndrome. (a) At the age of 2 years there is a trochanteric lesion through which a fracture subsequently occurred and was treated by internal fixation. (b) At three and a half years a further fracture has occurred below the plate. Note the rapid extension of the disease process

Pyknodysostosis behaves similarly as do the fractures of *Albers Schönberg's disease* (osteopetrosis) (*Figure 7.6*). Severe and progressive anaemia with cranial nerve entrapment may develop. *Generalized fibrous dysplasia* has a predilection for the trochanteric region and, if there is pain, this indicates that a crack fracture has occurred, usually through the calcar, and internal fixation by a nail plate is

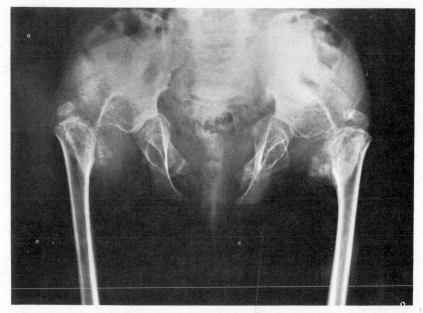

Figure 7.9. Severe coxa vara in spondylo-epiphyseal dysplasia congenita resembling dislocation but the head is visible opposite the acetabulum

needed. This may prevent displacement, but sometimes this develops in spite of fixation and the operation may need to be repeated together with an abduction osteotomy (*Figure 7.7*). The same problem may arise when there is an association with precocious puberty (Albright's syndrome) (*Figure 7.8*). *Hyperpituitarism* of spontaneous onset or therapeutically induced by growth hormone may predispose to displacement of the upper femoral epiphysis. The most severe variety of coxa vara is seen in *Spondylo-epiphyseal dysplasia congenita* (*Figure 7.9*).

3. Conditions simulating Perthes' disease

The commonest error is to confuse *Dysplasia multiplex epiphysealis* with bilateral Perthes' disease (*Figure 7.10*). Epiphyseal dysplasia affects many joints including the spine, where osteochondritic changes and moderate scoliosis may be seen. The lower radial and tibial epiphyses are triangular and the knee and shoulder joints are frequently malformed. Shortening of stature is common (we have learnt recently that this is also a feature of Perthes' disease) and the family history may be helpful. Degenerative joint disease develops in adult life but it is unlikely that we will be able to prevent this in the hip by containment osteotomy, for the pathogenesis is quite different. We will also remember the possibility of *Sickle cell anaemia*, (*Figure 7.29*); *Gaucher's disease* (*Figure 7.33*) and *Tricorhinophalangeal dysplasia* with which sparse hair, prominent nose and short fingers are associated.

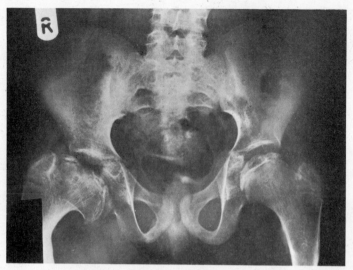

Figure 7.10. Dysplasia multiplex epiphysealis. (a) Note the resemblance to Perthes' disease.

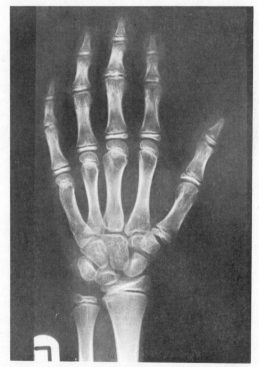

Figure 7.10. (b) The lower radial epiphysis is triangular

4. Dislocation of the hips

This dislocation, which is generally bilateral, is seen as a prominent feature in three conditions. In *Freeman–Sheldon syndrome* and its variations dislocations are associated with a pinched nose, ulnar deviation of the hand, congenital vertical talus and involvement of the knees. This is frequently misdiagnosed as arthrogryposis multiplex. The dislocated hips respond poorly to operative treatment because of their liability to stiffness and they should probably be left alone. *Diastrophic dwarfism (Figure 7.11)* displays the general features of

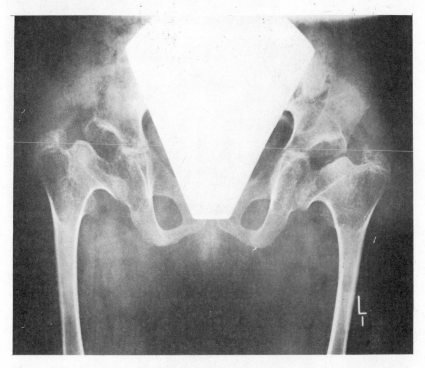

Figure 7.11. Diastrophic dwarfism. The hips are subluxated with deformity of the heads and severe acetabular dysplasia

achondroplasia with the addition of fixed deformities such as club feet, dislocated hips and flexed elbows. Cleft palate, cauliflower ears, and scoliosis are common. The hips resemble those of achondroplasia and are therefore malformed and best left untreated. Unlike achondroplasia, this is of recessive inheritance and the risk to further children is high. *Larsen's syndrome* describes a condition of multiple joint dislocations in which the hips share. Scoliosis, in the cervical spine especially, is common. The knees are dislocated into hyperextension and correction is likely to be at the expense of any pre-existing movement. The hips should therefore probably remain dislocated for fear of stiffness. This observation applies equally in other situations where knees and hips are involved in a generalized disorder.

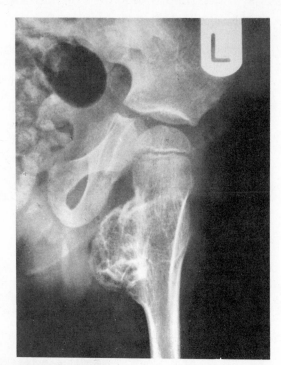

Figure 7.12. A trochanteric osteochondroma is associated with coxa valga. The hips will probably subluxate if this is not removed

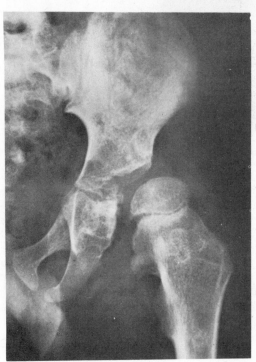

Figure 7.13. Cervical and acetabular osteochondromata have caused subluxation of the hip

236

5. Displacement of originally normal hips

An osteochondroma in *Diaphyseal aclasia* sometimes develops on the medial side of the trochanteric region and if it grows it will impinge against the pelvic wall, so displacing the femoral head laterally (*Figures 7.12, 7.13*). Removal is clearly indicated. The more proximal an osteochondroma, the more likely is malignant conversion, so that tumours in this area and the pelvis as a whole should be removed if growth is rapid. Peripheral osteochondromas are of little significance and may be excised if they cause symptoms, but sometimes the lower ulnar epiphysis closes prematurely leading to ulnar deviation of the hand, and the possibility of intraspinal tumours should not be forgotten. In *Dysplasia epiphysealis hemimelica* cartilaginous tumours arise within the epiphyses (*Figure 7.14*), most commonly at the knee and foot and, usually, unilaterally. Removal is indicated when they cause deformity or restrict movement. Although rare in the hip, this initially translucent tumour presents difficulty in diagnosis for the hip is likely to displace laterally without apparent cause. Later, the tumour may ossify in a patchy manner and declare its presence. Excision is indicated but the hip joint is likely to be damaged thereby. *Morquio's disease* may also progress to subluxation (*Figure 7.15*).

It is appropriate to mention *Juvenile rheumatoid arthritis* at this point. Although subluxation can usually be prevented by prompt diagnosis and good

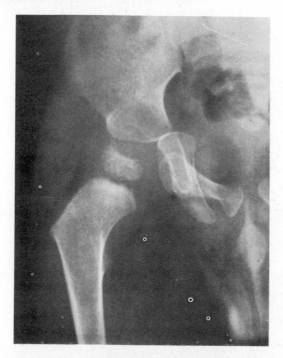

Figure 7.14. Dysplasia epiphysealis hemimelica. (a) The right hip is subluxated and there is a defect in the femoral head with some surrounding calcification

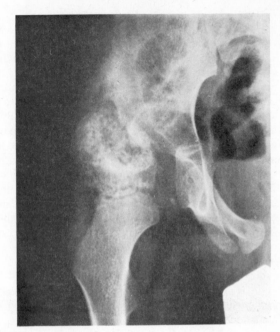

Figure 7.14. (b) Three years later the epiphyseal osteo-chondroma is evident

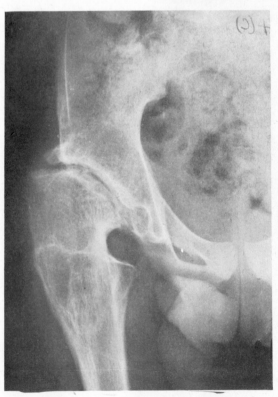

Figure 7.14. (c) Ten years later, following removal of the osteochondroma and varus osteotomy, the outcome is poor

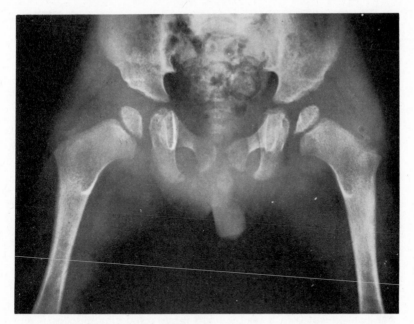

Figure 7.15. Morquio's disease. (a) At 2 years the hips are relatively normal

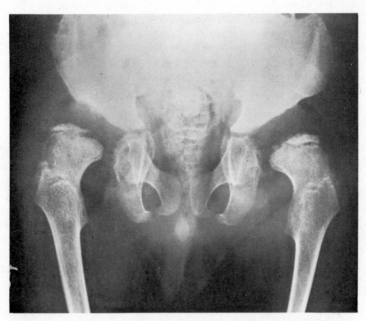

Figure 7.15. (b) At 7½ years lateral displacement and subluxation are evident

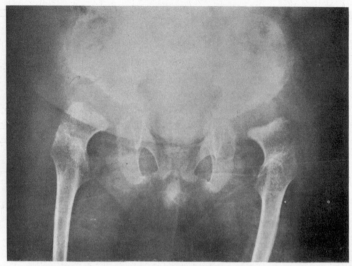

Figure 7.15. (c) At 12 years of age

general management (which for the joints means rest during episodes of activity and graduated movement during remissions), this complication is still sometimes seen when diagnosis is delayed and treatment is more sympathetic than effective. Delay in diagnosis is often due to the failure to appreciate that the onset may be before the age of 2 years and usually under 5 years, together with failure to examine all joints (especially the talocalcaneal) in all patients with mono-articular arthritis. When the vogue for cortisone was with us subluxation was sometimes caused and complicated by destructive erosion of the femoral head, but this is now rarely seen. Nonetheless, it is in this condition that we still occasionally find an indication for total replacement in the very young, especially when the knees are also involved and functional activity is greatly reduced.

6. Metaphyseal lesions

Rickets of varying type and their simulator metaphyseal dysostosis have already been mentioned. The generalized variety of *Histiocytosis* (Hand-Schueller-Christian) frequently involves the proximal femur and fractures may occur. Diabetes insipidus, dermatitis and pulmonary infiltration may complicate the situation. *Lead poisoning* may present as dense zones parallel to the growth plate, being wider the nearer they are to the plate. Anaemia, fits, and mental retardation, due to cerebral involvement, are serious associations. Somewhat similar appearances are seen in *Fluorosis* but they tend to be more diffuse. Such dense zones are not uncommonly seen in normal children and they tend to disappear with time. They may represent periods of arrested growth, although in situation and depth they differ from the more familiar Harris' lines. *Melorheostosis* is prone to involve part of the femoral head, calcar, and acetabulum in the well-recognized candle-wax fashion. Pain, contractures, shortening and scleroderma may be expected in varying degree.

7. The pelvis

Many of the conditions mentioned above also declare their presence in pelvic abnormalities, e.g. symphysis defect in craniocleidodysostosis, pelvic compression with diminished outlet in rickets and osteogenesis imperfecta (*Figure 7.5*), alternating iliac lines in osteopetrosis etc. The *Nail-Patella syndrome* displays the

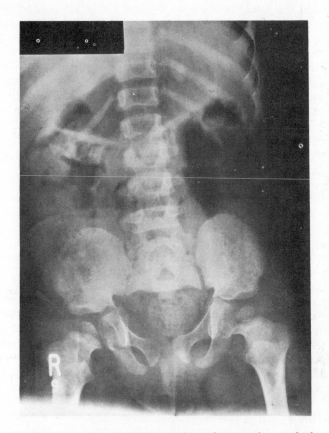

Figure 7.16. Achondroplasia. At this early stage the vertebral peduncles do not diverge in the lower lumbar spine

curious iliac horns which protrude posterolaterally and which are usually palpable. Dysplastic nails, hypoplasia of the patella, cubitus valgus and proteinuria, which may indicate a serious renal disorder, comprise the clinical features. The familiar *Achondroplasia* is characterized by a low broad pelvis and horizontal sacrum. The pelvic outlet is diminished and vaginal delivery is usually impossible. Spinal stenosis, due to reduction in the interpeduncular distance within the lumbar spine, is very rarely seen in children but hydrocephalus secondary to narrowing of the foramen magnum may develop (*Figure 7.16*).

B. SUNDRY DISORDERS OF THE SOFT TISSUES

Arthrogryposis multiplex congenita

In this disorder the hips are frequently affected by either deformity (especially fixed flexion and abduction) or dislocation. Fixed deformity is usually secondary to knee flexion, which imposes flexion and abduction on the hip when the baby lies supine or prone. Sometimes however, both are seen in company with fixed extension of the knee. In either event these deformities, unlike most in this condition, frequently respond to stretching, especially if flexed knees are corrected and the child is nursed prone. Operation to release soft tissues is fortunately seldom necessary for there is a tendency to myositis ossificans.

The management of dislocation is the essential consideration. When there is fixed flexion in infancy it may be difficult to decide whether dislocation is present but there is no immediate urgency and the true situation will be revealed as deformity relaxes. When present, dislocations are most likely to be complete and bilateral. Operative reduction is almost invariably necessary and the techniques employed are similar to those used in simple congenital dislocation. We should not, however, expect the outcome to be as favourable despite a satisfactory anatomical reposition, for any initial stiffness is likely to increase.

The selection of patients for surgical treatment demands careful consideration, for persistent dislocation may add little to the total handicap in a severely-affected child, whereas reduction with further loss of movement may well contribute to the disability. It is probably prudent to deny reduction if there is persistent flexion deformity and a flexion range of less than 90° with a comparable loss of abduction. An exception may be made if only one hip is dislocated and the other is mobile, stable and well controlled (*Figure 7.17*). There is a further fundamental factor in selection, namely the strength not only of the hip musculature but of the child as a whole. A useful clinical classification of arthrogryposis divides the patients into the weak and the strong. That this variability should arise is not surprising if we regard arthrogryposis as a syndrome which represents the final common path of arrested intra-uterine myopathy or neuropathy. Although some muscles are absent or fibrotic and non-functioning, the remainder are present and must be assessed for power. General weakness neutralizes the benefits of surgical correction and the child is likely to become confined to a chair. Some patients have selective weakness which commonly involves the arms predominantly with relative sparing of the legs, while still others may have strong hip musculature but are virtually paralyzed below the knees. Such considerations are clearly vital to the process of selection, for general or selective hip weakness will contra-indicate reduction. There are two further implications. Firstly, we should postpone our decision until the child can be accurately assessed which may mean a delay of up to two years. Intelligence is very seldom impaired and indeed is frequently high. Secondly, when arms are virtually useless the feet may take over the functions of hands, which requires that there be hypermobility in the joints of the legs, to which dislocated hips make a useful contribution (Lloyd-Roberts and Lettin, 1970).

Joint laxity

This has been mentioned as a factor in the aetiology and management of congenital dislocation together with the hypotonia with which it is so often associated. In

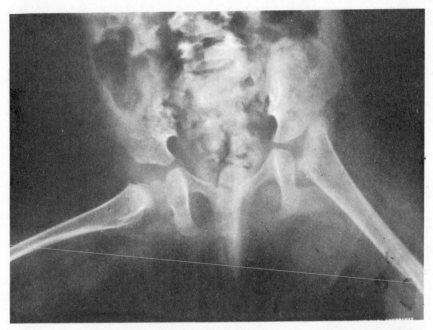

Figure 7.17. Arthrogryposis. (a) The left hip is dislocated but the right is stable and mobile

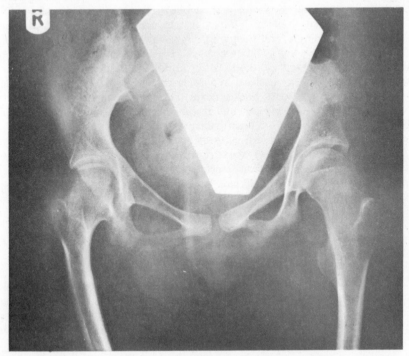

Figure 7.17. (b) Eleven years after open reduction on the left

243

combination these are the commonest cause of moderate delay in walking which may extend to the second birthday, especially when the child discovers the potential of bottom-crawling. This is usually benign and self-limiting and there are no permanent effects. Persistence beyond the age of 2 years will alert the clinician to the possibility of an identifiable underlying cause. By this age, the ability to abduct the flexed hips to 90° should arouse suspicion. Some will declare themselves as one or other variety of congenital myotonia with a varying severity and prognosis which spans the spectrum from persistent non-progressive hypotonia with perhaps some deformity (Oppenheimer's disease of earlier terminology) to progressive spinal-cord degeneration (Werdnig-Hoffman disease). Knowledge of these myopathic and neuropathic disorders is developing rapidly as diagnostic precision improves as a result of more sophisticated electromyographic techniques and the histochemical examination of biopsy specimens together with enzyme assay of the peripheral blood. It is essential that the surgeon be aware of the true nature of these disorders for the diagnosis of a progressive variety will usually contra-indicate surgical treatment.

Persistent joint laxity may also suggest certain other syndromes with which it is associated. In *Mental deficiency* of a degree which considerably delays walking, hypotonia combines with delay to modify the appearance of the hips. The femoral necks are long and vertical, with less than normal acetabular cover so that dysplasia is often suspected (*Figure 7.23*). *Ehlers–Danlos syndrome* is characterized by friable, over-stretchable skin and severe laxity and is of autosomal inheritance. Laxity is largely responsible for the disability which may present at birth as congenital dislocation of the hips or later, when other joints suffer recurrent dislocation. Scoliosis may develop (Beighton and Horan, 1969). Laxity and subluxation of the hip may also appear in association with *Marfan's disease* (arachnodactyly) and *Homocystinuria*, which once again include scoliosis among the manifestations (Brenton *et al.*, 1972). Laxity is also a feature of several general disorders of the skeleton of which *Osteogenesis imperfecta* is the most familiar. There is also a hypotonic variety of *Cerebral palsy* in which weakness is associated with brisk reflexes. This may be the result of a specific pattern of brain injury and athetoid features frequently emerge later. Alternatively, the primary cause of brain damage may be severe hypotonia which is responsible for respiratory difficulty at birth. Lastly there is a *Familial type* (Carter and Wilkinson, 1964) of laxity with little if any hypotonia. Recurrent dislocation of joints is common, especially the patella, and posterior displacement of the shoulder. This may be a factor in congenital dislocation of the hip, especially in boys; more commonly, the femoral head is at first seen to stand away from a normal acetabulum but the joint develops satisfactorily later.

Calcification and ossification

Discrete areas of calcification are sometimes seen in the necrotic muscle bundles of *Myositis and Dermatomyositis* but they are unusual around the hip in children. In *Haemophilia* also, the forearm and calf are much commoner than the hip. Similarly *Tumoral calcinosis* favours the elbow. In *Dysplasia epiphysealis punctata* (stippled epiphyses) calcification may spread to periarticular structures.

B. SUNDRY DISORDERS OF THE SOFT TISSUES

Myositis ossificans, however, is not infrequently seen in the region of the hip. This may on occasion be the result of local injury — surgical or accidental. Children with spastic paraplegia seem less prone than adults to myositis ossificans, but this complication is uncommon in children with cerebral palsy. *Familial myositis ossificans progressiva (Figure 7.18)* frequently involves the hip musculature when sheets of well-differentiated bone replace muscle and cause, at first,

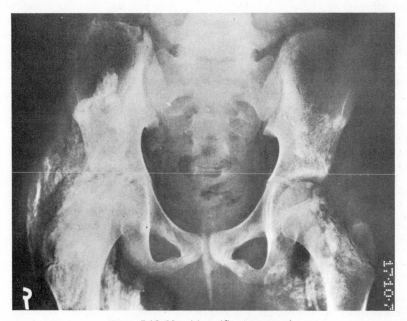

Figure 7.18. Myositis ossificans progressiva

limitation of movement and, later, fixed deformity. The familial nature is shown in the short first metatarsals and metacarpals. At the onset, brawny tender swellings around the shoulder girdle ossify progressively, causing later a life-threatening loss of respiratory movement. Removal of troublesome bony bars should if possible be delayed until their structure suggests that they are composed of mature bone. Even then, recurrence is all too common in spite of the use of corticosteroids (Harris, 1961).

Progressive myositis may be due to *repeated injections* and is therefore likely to involve the thigh and buttocks. It is a sad commentary on our time that this has been seen in a 17-year-old youth already addicted to drugs.

Therapeutic injections in the neonatal period may also be responsible, but contracture of gluteus medius is more commonly seen. Unlike the corresponding contracture in the quadriceps (Gunn, 1964; Lloyd-Roberts and Thomas, 1964), this usually responds to stretching. Idiopathic contracture is also a possibility but both this and congenital absence of muscle is rare in the pelvic as opposed to the shoulder girdle.

245

Diffuse soft tissue tumours

When the thigh shares in an overall gigantism of the limb we may suspect neuro-fibromatosis, fibro-fatty overgrowth, diffuse cavernous haemangiomata or multiple congenital arteriovenous fistulae to be the cause. All are associated with abnormalities of form, thus distinguishing them from the normal profile of simple hemihypertrophy. *Neurofibromatosis* of this type is usually associated with stigmata of the disease elsewhere and it is probable that the bones will display variation in length, girth and contour. The hyperplasia of nerve sheaths, amounting sometimes to plexiform neuromata, is sometimes painful and, together with deformity, may indicate amputation. The pain may obscure the onset of sarcomatous metaplasia. *Diffuse cavernous haemangioma* is a potentially dangerous condition for recurrent haemorrhage within the vascular spaces overstresses the body's capacity to replace platelets so that thrombocytopaenia and, in consequence, a tendency to further haemorrhage develops. Amputation may be needed to save life. Muscle contractures and arthropathy due to recurrent haemorrhages add to the problems. *Arteriovenous fistulae* are multiple and are characterized by venous congestion, warmth of the leg and audible bruits. The pulse pressure is raised and if cardiac failure develops amputation may be necessary. Most, however, are less threatening in their presentation and, as in superficial diffuse angiomatous malformation, leg-shortening operations are often of benefit. Attempts to ligate the fistulae are always unrewarding (others will promptly open up) and often disastrous if free venous return is compromised or the distal part of the limb is short-circuited.

Localized neoplasms

These include haemangio-lipoma, diffuse infiltrating angioma and fibroblastic tumours. Primary fibro-sarcomas, rhabdomyosarcomas of voluntary muscle and malignant synoviomas may, on account of their rarity in children, be omitted from this discussion. *Haemangiolipoma* has a special predilection for the front of the thigh where it is often overlooked until haemorrhage causes pain and draws attention to the lump. At operation it is poorly defined in relation to surrounding fat but local, if incomplete, excision relieves the symptom. *Diffuse infiltrating angiomas* favour the pelvic area and in their nature are difficult to eradicate completely. The residium may be radiosensitive. The *fibroblastic (desmoid) group* of tumours are particularly prone to the gluteal region. In their clinical presentation they simulate fibrosarcoma, being hard, fixed to deeper structures, and often crossed by dilated veins. They do not metastasize nor do they invade, but expand proximally in muscle planes so that they soon enter the sciatic notch. The sciatic nerve transmits normally in spite of infiltration of the tumour between the nerve bundles. This feature will make local excision without sacrifice of the nerve impractical and we then have two alternatives. If pain is a prominent feature hemipelvectomy is the only recourse but, if not, we may wait in the hope that tumour growth will be slower than that of the patient and will cease at maturity. The histological distinction between fibrosarcoma and fibroblastic tumour can be very testing, and indeed the subsequent clinical course may be the ultimate differentiation. Whether fibrosarcomatous change represents metaplasia in a pre-existing fibroblastic tumour or whether this co-existed throughout in an area which was not examined histologically is uncertain. Fibrosarcoma is rare unless the fibroblastic tumour has been irradiated. Two personal cases of sarcomatous degeneration had been exposed to irradiation.

C. NEUROLOGICAL DISEASES

1. Cerebral palsy

Management in all patients depends upon careful assessment of intellectual, emotional, physical and prognostic factors. However here we will assume that the child as a whole is suitable for treatment and consider the purely technical aspects of deformity and displacement of the hips.

Deformity is generally flexion or adduction or a combination of both which may be associated with subluxation or dislocation of the hip. Less commonly, internal rotation is a significant feature, being superimposed upon adduction. These deformities may be dynamic, being present only on walking or on clinical examination and disappearing during sleep and under anaesthesia or fixed by structural adaptation. The distinction is important for splinting alone is unlikely to influence fixed deformity and attempts at correction by manual stretching will dishearten the physiotherapist. Dynamic deformity, on the other hand, may frequently be reduced, if not overcome, by such methods and, perhaps more significantly, may be prevented from becoming structural.

Deformity in this context does not necessarily mean fixed deformity in the sense that the opposite movement is abolished. Thus, hip adduction is more frequently associated with limited abduction rather than with failure to achieve the neutral position when the range of passive movement is estimated. We are more concerned with the posture adopted on walking which, if consistent, i.e. adduction and internal rotation, constitutes a functional fixed deformity whatever the passive range. Careful observation of gait together with an assessment of performance, estimated by the time taken to cover a given distance, are the most important clinical features. Assessment of deformity, loss of movement, spasm and power in the resting condition follow but are of secondary significance.

In our analysis of gait we observe not only the walking posture of the hip but also that of the leg as a whole. Thus, severe calf spasm leading to marked equinus may cause knee and hip flexion on walking when in fact the hip has no intrinsic limitation of movement. Adduction and internal rotation are likely to be the most conspicuous features and are seen in isolation or combination. Adduction may be associated with a lurching gait due either to apparent shortening or to weakness and inhibition of the abductors. If combined with internal rotation, the leg may obstruct the forward step of a normal limb in hemiplegia or prevent walking altogether when the knees are compressed together in diplegia. Subluxation or dislocation will aggravate the problem. Lastly, short steps may be due to shortening of the hamstrings. Although deformity, loss of movement, and hip-joint displacement will, for convenience, be considered separately it should be appreciated that they are seldom present either in isolation or in the absence of distal primary or secondary changes in the same limb or, in the event of diplegia, on the opposite side.

Fixed hip flexion is frequently seen in association with flexed knees and is secondary to this. If, when conscious, the child lies supine with flexed knees this inevitably imposes a flexion attitude on the hips. During sleep adductor spasm relaxes and the child, if supine, lies in a frog-like position in which once again the hips are flexed. In these circumstances dynamic flexion rapidly becomes structural; but, by the same token, correction is equally rapid if the cause is removed. If the knees are straightened, and plaster tubes with a cross-bar are applied, and the child lies prone, the hip deformity will usually respond rapidly. Although this principle may be successfully applied at almost any age, it is of course more likely to succeed in the young, for some older children develop a deformity which resists non-surgical correction. Formal soft-tissue correction is therefore sometimes necessary, for correction by traction, although occasionally profitable, is likely to be followed by relapse if the deforming dynamic forces remain uncorrected. The operation involves release of all tight structures in front of the joint and this may include the capsule. The psoas if contracted must certainly be divided or transplanted laterally when abductor weakness, adduction deformity, or spasm are prominent features. It is of course essential to correct adduction contracture. Osteotomy in the growing child is unnecessary and, indeed, ineffective if the deforming forces remain unimpaired. At skeletal maturity however, this is sometimes indicated especially when adduction and rotational deformities are associated, but once again the soft tissues should not be ignored because of the dynamic effect of persisting spasm when walking is resumed.

Correction of adduction on walking is certainly our most frequent concern. Physical methods and splinting applied intermittently are unlikely to be of benefit if the child habitually walks in adduction. Furthermore, such a gait exposes the hip to the risk of subluxation. Tenotomy alone is inadequate for we must both release structural contracture and weaken the muscles if recurrence is to be prevented. We must certainly divide adductor longus and gracilis and sometimes even part of adductor brevis and magnus if abduction is still restricted. The anterior branch of the obturator nerve lying upon the anterior surface of adductor brevis is also divided. If fixed flexion deformity is significant, exposure may be deepened to divide the iliopsoas tendon by dissection between adductor brevis and pectineus. A further refinement in this circumstance is to transplant the adductors to the ischial tuberosity (Stephenson and Donovan, 1969), a technique which is the subject of encouraging reports. Following tenotomy and neurectomy, a double hip spica is applied for no more than 3 weeks to prevent the pelvis from tilting, which would reduce the correction obtained. Thereafter, stretching by physiotherapist and parents starts again. Unfortunately recurrence is not unknown because of either the failure to persist with stretching or continuing imbalance between adductors and greatly weakened abductors. We must once again divide adductor contractures and consider transplantation of iliopsoas to the greater trochanter to reinforce abductor power.

Internal rotation is frequently associated with adduction, especially in diplegia when it adds to the disability by causing the feet to cross one another. Relief of the adduction element will often overcome this problem by increasing the distance between the ankles, but sometimes it persists as a specific functional handicap especially if flexion remains uncorrected. In the young child some benefit may follow transplantation of the semitendinosus to the lateral femoral condyle. This muscle, in company with the adductors, is under increased tension if the hip is flexed, since both combine as internal rotators. Recession of the anterior half of gluteus medius with the tensor fascia femoris by folding them backwards over the posterior segment and securing them to the iliac crest is sometimes recommended. These muscles are internal rotators but, from my limited experience, little advantage is gained by their recession and it may be that some relief of flexion is responsible for such advantage as there is. In older children torsion of the femur, especially anteversion of the neck, establishes the deformity and operations on muscles are unavailing. It is essential to confirm or deny structural rotation by examination under anaesthesia, and to proceed to osteotomy if this is present. Rotation osteotomy should be performed below the lesser trochanter for, if intertrochanteric, the insertion of psoas is displaced forwards thus augmenting its power as an internal rotator.

Although *Extension contracture* is not seen, limitation of hip flexion may be due to hamstring contracture. This is particularly evident in diplegia as a cause of knee flexion on walking and is one of the indications for transplanting the hamstrings to the femur. Less commonly, the gait is characterized by short steps with straight knees and straight leg-raising may be reduced to less than 45°. This is well described by Seymour and Sharrard (1968) who have developed an operation to detach the origin of the hamstrings from the ischial tuberosity, which is of value in this situation.

Subluxation and dislocation are acquired rather than congenital and they can usually be prevented if the surgeon is alert to the possibility. This is a most undesirable complication for not only is instability superadded but it becomes more difficult to control flexion and adduction, pain may intrude later and in hemiplegia there is shortening which is both true and apparent due to an increase in pelvic obliquity. The mechanism is similar to that in myelomeningocele and poliomyelitis, namely an imbalance in power and length between flexors and adductors which are dislocating forces and the abductors and extensors which are the stabilizers (Sharrard, 1971). There are also other contributory factors such as femoral anteversion and valgus (Samilson *et al.,* 1972), and rarely, scoliosis. Muscle imbalance however would seem to be the prime factor for reduction, stabilized by osteotomy alone, is likely to be followed by redislocation if the imbalance remains uncorrected.

Prevention implies detection of minor subluxation by annual radiographic control of all patients in whom adductor and flexor involvement is present. There is then an immediate indication for adductor tenotomy and anterior obturator neurectomy, coupled with psoas tenotomy through the same incision, if flexion spasm or deformity is significant. The same operation may be used when subluxation is more pronounced, providing that congruity is restored with the legs in neutral position when examined under anaesthesia — once this point is passed subluxation will usually progress even to the extent of dislocation. A varus and lateral rotation osteotomy will then be necessary in addition to adductor and flexor release. The gradual development of displacement has two advantages. Firstly, it is unusual to have to perform a formal open reduction for, generally, congruity is restored when anteversion and valgus are corrected. Secondly, the relatively late onset means that the acetabulum has been stimulated by a contained head for some years so that its development is usually satisfactory. Furthermore, this is not inhibited by the genetic influences which may operate in congenital dislocation (*Figure 7.19*).

Osteotomy, necessary though it is, may introduce new problems. The external rotation component can be only advantageous for it also corrects any tendency to internal rotation. The varus element however may reduce abductor power by shortening the distance between muscle origin and insertion. We should therefore

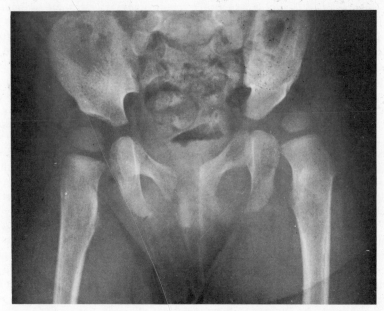

Figure 7.19. Cerebral palsy. The hip is subluxating and requires surgical treatment

make radiological studies pre-operatively in abduction and internal rotation alone in the hope that a subtrochanteric rotation osteotomy without varus will accomplish our objective. If varus is necessary we should consider lateral transplantation of iliopsoas rather than tenotomy or, as an alternative, distal advancement of the greater trochanter.

We must now consider the surgical *Relief of pain* when analgesics are unavailing, and the *Maintenance of cleanliness* in the bed-ridden. Pain is a rare feature of subluxation and dislocation in the walking patient but, when present, it is a formidable problem. It is due to secondary osteoarthritis, aggravated by the muscle spasm of the underlying disease, augmented by reflex spasm secondary to arthritis. Surgery has little if anything to offer and we must depend upon analgesics, walking sticks, crutches and finally a wheelchair. Those already restricted to a wheelchair may also suffer, especially if dislocation is associated with the involuntary movements of athetosis. Excision of the head and neck of the femur will relieve the pain, but at the price of some discomfort due to movement of the great trochanter beneath the skin. Lastly, we not infrequently meet a severely retarded and bedridden child who is usually quadriplegic with severe adductor spasm. Cleanliness is the major management problem which radical open adductor tenotomy and division of both branches of the obturator nerve will resolve.

C. NEUROLOGICAL DISEASES

2. Myelomeningocele

Considerable energy has been directed in recent years towards the treatment of residual peripheral paralysis and much of this concerns the correction of instability and deformity of the hips. The subject has been comprehensively reviewed by Sharrard (1971) and Menelaus (1971), to whom the reader is referred for detailed information; only the general principles of management will be outlined here.

There has recently been a notable tendency among those responsible for the primary care of the newborn to become selective in their use of life-saving measures such as urgent closure of the sac and immediate drainage of hydrocephalus. The result is that the number of children surviving to an age when reconstructive surgery merits consideration have not only greatly decreased but also commonly have a neurological defect distal to the L.4 segment which offers the surgeon some prospect of benefitting the child. Laurence (1964) studied the natural history of untreated babies and found that 70 per cent died within three years — most within the first year. When treated the mortality is 40 per cent, but in both groups of survivors the intellectual, physical and sphincteric disturbance was comparable. The prospect for those living beyond the age of 3 years is that approximately half will have the mental and physical capacity to attend a normal school but this must surely largely apply to treated patients for we do not for practical purposes see untreated patients surviving at the age when schooling normally begins. As a result of selective treatment, therefore, overall survival is greatly reduced and of those patients living to school age a higher proportion probably will be equipped to attend.

The ability to attend primary school does not mean that the adult will be able to earn his living independently. Several factors contribute to this — physical, emotional and sociological. Physically, increasing weight, amounting often to gross obesity, coupled with sensory loss and often scoliosis, may make the ordeal of walking intolerable and a wheelchair is preferred. There may be some intellectual impairment and this, with the demoralization which the realization of their plight so often brings about, contributes to their decision to abandon the effort. In combination, these influences are generally apparent at the age of 12 to 14 years. Lastly, whether walking with difficulty or not, employment opportunities are very limited. There are few residential sheltered workshops so that for most there is the problem of travelling to work and, even if this is possible, finding that their limited capabilities are more efficiently and economically replaced by machines. In days of economic stringency, few employers can afford for humanitarian reasons to make their industry more labour-intensive than it need be.

In considering treatment of the hips, we must constantly be aware of these disquieting facts and resist the temptation to indulge in surgical adventures which, even if successful in the short term, contribute little to the wellbeing of the older child or adult.

Indications

Fixed flexion deformity, subluxation, and dislocation are our main concern but other deformities sometimes require consideration. Thus external rotation and abduction or adduction sometimes compromise caliper-fitting or walking and

MISCELLANEOUS

require soft-tissue release or, on occasion, osteotomy for rotation. Lumbar scoliosis will not only encourage dislocation but, if severe, may sometimes indicate fusion to improve the sitting balance but seldom if ever to stabilize a dislocation. If scoliosis is mild or moderate, varus osteotomy with psoas transplantation and contralateral abductor release may be helpful.

Fixed flexion with or without displacement of the hip is the major problem and this is due to the unopposed action of flexors and adductors. This combination of deformity and dislocation is almost inevitable when paralysis spares the L.4 segment but less common when L.5 is spared and some abductor power is preserved. Similarly lesions above L.1 affect the adductors and dislocation is a less conspicuous feature.

Fixed flexion is almost constant at birth unless the psoas is paralyzed at the thoracic level and even then flexion imposed by uterine posture may be present. Subluxation and dislocation may be evident at birth or occur later because of muscle imbalance. Most of the deaths occur within the first year, so major surgery is best avoided during this time which may be usefully spent in assessment, muscle-charting and stretching of deformity. Splinting of the hip which reduces easily is of little value for dislocation will recur when the splint is removed and trophic ulceration may be a complication. At 1 year any residual and significant flexion and adduction should be corrected for these will compromise caliper-fitting and walking, and if corrected there will be no interference with sitting if a wheelchair is the final outcome. Adduction presents no great difficulty for open tenotomy, extended as necessary to obtain full abduction, will not compromise later treatment of dislocation, whereas incidental psoas tenotomy for flexion will prevent its transplantation later. It is therefore essential to decide now whether or not to treat hip displacement if it is present.

The presence of dislocation or subluxation is not in itself an indication to reduce and stabilize the hips. For example, in high lesions with sparing of flexors and adductors alone the outcome is so poor that no more than release of deforming contractures is necessary. Preservation of some or good quadriceps power when L.4 is spared does not greatly modify the outcome, for lack of hip extension (posterior psoas transplantation notwithstanding) will dictate the use of calipers with pelvic band, or if no band then long-leg calipers and a walking-frame or clumpers. In contrast when L.5 is spared, useful function may be obtained and maintained so that reduction and stabilization are indicated. Unilateral dislocation at almost any level of paralysis should however be treated to control deformity and as an aid to caliper-fitting. Subluxation in low lesions indicates operation to prevent dislocation but in high lesions the inevitable subsequent dislocation should be accepted. It should be remembered that these children are likely to revert to a wheelchair in early adolescence and are not therefore, handicapped by flexion deformity and do not suffer painful arthritis later in life.

Treatment

This is usually directed towards correction of *Flexion and adduction deformities* and only sometimes reduction of subluxation and dislocation. Both adduction and flexion may respond to simple stretching, especially when deformity is postural, and is a reflection of the intra-uterine position imposed upon a flail hip. In such patients we commonly see a combination of knee and hip flexion and the child lies in this position. As in cerebral palsy, if the knees are corrected and maintained in plaster cylinders with a cross-bar and the child lies prone, hip flexion will frequently disappear. If however the dynamic force of muscle imbalance is the responsible agent, operation is generally necessary to complete the correction. Radical open adductor tenotomy may be combined with division of the psoas tendon through the same incision. It is unusual to follow this with an anterior release unless, in the flail, abduction has caused a contracture of tensor fascia femoris. Osteotomy is best avoided in the early years for it is seldom possible to neutralize completely the imbalance and recurrence is then probable. It should certainly never be performed without attention to the soft tissues.

When *Subluxation or dislocation* are to be treated it is equally essential that muscle imbalance or contracture be corrected or redislocation will certainly occur. Although on occasion we may treat a unilateral dislocation in a relatively flail hip by adductor release, reduction and varus osteotomy coupled with division of the psoas, it is usually preferable to transplant the psoas laterally. The transplant not only permanently removes a deforming force but, by harnessing an innervated muscle as an activated tenodesis, we reinforce the stability of the reduction. The term 'activated tenodesis' is used for it is very doubtful whether the transplanted muscle ever functions in a controlled fashion during that phase in walking (extension) which is diametrically opposed to that for which it has evolved (flexion). The tendon may be inserted laterally to provide an abducting tether (Mustard, 1959), or posteriorly when it has an extending effect (Sharrard, 1964). Both methods are, with few exceptions, effective in preventing redislocation but Sharrard expects to reduce the length of the caliper to below hip level if his posterior transplant is used (Carroll and Sharrard, 1972). The lateral transplant is however an easier operation in that less intrapelvic mobilization is needed and the new attachment of the psoas is likely to be more secure. If long-standing flexion deformity has caused shortening of the psoas, it may be difficult to obtain the length needed for secure fixation posteriorly, whereas there is ample tendon available for a lateral insertion (*Figure 7.20*).

The operative steps used as preliminaries to either transplant are variable. Adductor release is essential and any residual flexion is coincidentally corrected by the extensive anterior exposure. It is seldom necessary to perform a formal open reduction as in congenital dislocation nor to realign or deepen the acetabulum, for congruous reduction is usually achieved by positioning alone once contractures have been released. The position of greatest stability in relation to the neutral will decide the need or otherwise for concurrent varus and external rotation femoral osteotomy, which is certainly not indicated as a routine. The capsule should be opened not only to confirm the quality of reduction but also to excise redundant capsule and plicate the remainder for added stability.

Certain alternatives have been attempted without success. Lorenz's bifurcation osteotomy, when dislocation is accepted and deformity is paramount, has no advantage over soft-tissue release for no increased stability is obtained thereby. Colonna's arthroplasty may be followed by neuropathic changes, and psoas translocation, in which the psoas is passed behind the neck of the femur with its continuity maintained, develops so much tension that flexion is restricted and the knee hyperextends.

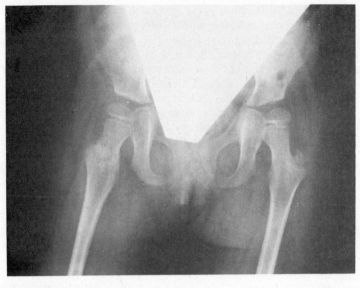

(a)

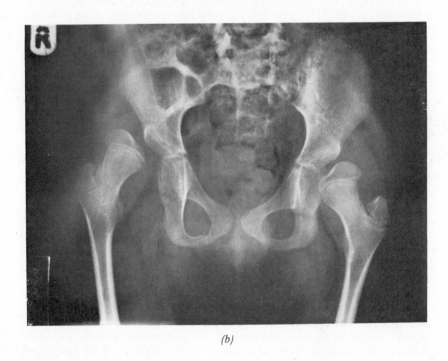

(b)

Figure 7.20. The hips in myelomeningocele. (a) At 5 years both hips are stable. (b) At 10 years the right is dislocated and the left subluxated

254

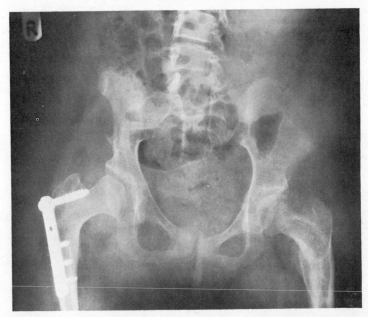

Figure 7.20. (c) Following open reduction, psoas transplantation and femoral osteotomy on the right and osteotomy with division of adductors and psoas on the left

There remain a few *General observations*. Firstly, it is fruitless to attempt caliper-walking before the age of 2 years and often this is only achieved even later. Secondly, postoperative greenstick supracondylar fractures are commonplace due to the porosis of paralysis and immobility. A Jones bandage is usually sufficient because the fractures are stable and painless. If urinary diversion is to be performed the hips should, if possible, be dealt with first. Absorbable skin sutures should always be avoided for contamination with urine seems to cause their premature disintegration. Special care must always be used in applying plaster spicas in case sacral compression is followed by ulceration. Similarly, no force should be imposed on the limbs if plaster is used to maintain an operative or manipulative correction of deformity. Lastly, myelomeningocele is a condition which affects not only the limbs but also the renal tract and the central and spinal nervous system. The renal tract requires regular surveillance, the bowel must be trained and one must be mindful of the possibilities of deterioration due to recurring hydrocephalus, ascending gliosis of the spinal cord (sometimes with spasticity), psychological factors, and obesity.

3. Anterior poliomyelitis

Although this is a disappearing disease in developed countries there remain some areas of the world where, for administrative reasons, protection is not available before children first attend school. Thus we still see some patients for whose condition the synonym infantile paralysis is appropriate. The pathogenesis and natural history are well described in the literature of the first half of this century, and there is a recent review by Sharrard (1971) which summarizes our knowledge. We, however, will merely consider somewhat superficially the features of residual paralysis as they affect the hip.

If extension, preferably with some abductor power, is retained the hip will ₁₀main stable and the child will walk without artificial aid even if totally paralyzed distally, providing that there is some equinus at the ankle and no flexion deformity

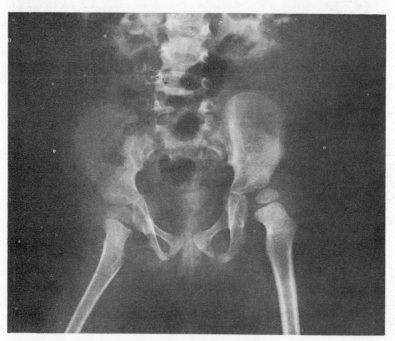

Figure 7.21. Poliomyelitis. There is an abduction contracture on the right which has caused the unaffected left hip to subluxate

of the knee. This is because active extension in the stance phase of walking imposes a hyperextension force on the knee which locks in this position. Hyper-extension is augmented by equinus at the ankle and stabilized by contact of the foot with the ground. In order to capitalize on this we must frequently correct knee flexion deformity and establish equinus if this is not already present. At the knee in the young child, soft-tissue release (avoiding capsulotomy in case excessive recurvation develops) and serial plaster correction is usually sufficient, provided that stretching, and often splinting at night, is continued for several years. Later, osteotomy with deliberate, but very limited, hyperextension is preferable. Similarly the Achilles tendon may be shortened early and arthrodesis of the ankle substituted later.

Correction of knee flexion will almost invariably include division of tensor fascia femoris (fascia lata) for contracture therein is a common and most important aspect not only of this but also of the final pattern of deformity. Unrelieved contracture may cause flexion and posterior subluxation of the knee together with lateral rotation of the tibia. The hip is abducted and flexed but one deformity may obscure the other if not specifically sought. Thus, if the child lies with hip abducted, flexion may be masked, and if flexion is detected, abduction may be overlooked unless the hip is adducted with as little flexion as is possible. The pelvic obliquity so produced has certain implications. Firstly, while it helps to stabilize the ipsolateral hip, it exposes the contralateral to the risk of dislocation (*Figure 7.21*). Secondly, flexion deformity will inhibit any residual extensor activity. Lastly, it causes scoliosis of the lumbar spine. Correction is indicated and involves proximal, and sometimes distal, transverse division of the fascia lata, occasionally reinforced, in the interests of residual flexion, by a release of the hip flexor muscles from the pelvis and psoas from the femur. Osteotomy is rarely necessary. The release should not be overenthusiastic and correction should not amount to the restoration of free adduction in extension for then the hip may lose some of the stability which some abduction provides. Furthermore, if there is associated spinal muscle paralysis which will potentiate the lumbar scoliosis, we must not forget the value of transplanting tensor fascia femoris with a segment of gluteus maximus to the lower ribs (Axer, 1958) as an alternative to tenotomy.

Subluxation and dislocation are caused by imbalance between flexors and adductors on the one hand and abductors and extensors on the other. Pelvic obliquity as already mentioned may reduce or augment the risk. The situation is similar to that seen in myelomeningocele, for dislocation does not occur when hips are flail nor when some abductor power remains. Hip displacement is unusual if the disease is contracted after the age of 2 years (Parsons and Seddon, 1968), although an ischial-bearing caliper may predispose in older children. Predisposing contractures must be released and this, as already indicated, may be abduction and flexion of the opposite hip or adduction and flexion of the displaced hip. Congruity and stability will be restored in most if operation is not unduly delayed. In neglected patients, however, femoral varus osteotomy may be necessary to stabilize reduction in the weight-bearing position.

Psoas transplantation to the great trochanter was introduced by Mustard (1959) as a method of further stabilizing reduction and, in some circumstances, to improve the unstable gait of abductor weakness. He emphasized that not only must the psoas be unaffected but also that there should be some residual extensor power (MRC Scale 3) and, preferably, some sparing of the abductors. With this pattern of paralysis the operation is of great value providing that all surrounding contractures have been relieved and any residual incongruity of the hip has been corrected by osteotomy.

4. The floppy baby syndrome

This embracing term is used to describe a variety of neuropathic, myopathic and spinal or cerebral atrophies. These vary greatly in their outlook and it is essential that in spite of the difficulties an attempt is made to make an accurate diagnosis before treatment begins. Those of delayed onset such as pseudohypertrophic atrophy do not greatly concern us but the congenital myopathies may present

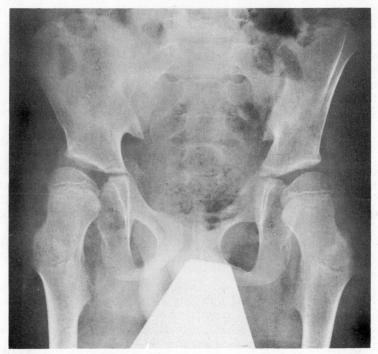

Figure 7.22. Congenital myopathy. This child had never walked and the hips, show the characteristic femoral valgus and anteversion with some subluxation

with either hip deformity or dislocation (*Figure 7.22*). An association with knee or foot deformity should however alert the surgeon, for with the exception of talipes calcaneus, 'idiopathic' hip dislocation is an isolated anomaly. Even the benign variety of hypotonia with joint laxity may cause problems. Delay in walking and persistence of infantile anteversion and valgus may cause subluxation which merits treatment (*Figure 7.23*). After operation, if the femur rolls into excessive external rotation, the hip may displace forwards. At the other end of the spectrum, Werdnig-Hoffman's progressive spinal atrophy will contra-indicate any treatment to the hips. In this difficult field the help of a paediatrically-orientated neurologist is essential and investigations will often include myelography, muscle-creatinine and enzyme assay, electromyography, and muscle biopsy before a decision can be made.

D. ROTATIONAL DEFORMITIES OF THE FEMUR

(a) Anteversion

The child presents with an in-toeing gait and because the medial rotation which causes this is situated above the knees the patellae will point more medially than usual. On examination in the supine position with the hips extended medial rotation of the hips will be increased at the expense of lateral rotation. When

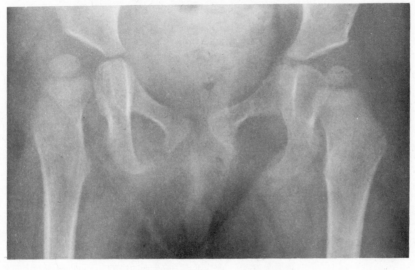

(a)

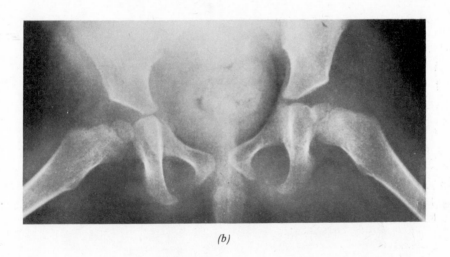

(b)

Figure 7.23. Hypotonia. (a) The right hip is subluxating in a child who has not walked by the age of 2 years. (b) Congruity is restored in abduction and internal rotation

the child is examined prone with extended hips and flexed knees, the tibia may be used as a protractor to measure the rotational discrepancy with greater accuracy. If the hips are flexed the difference is less and this is probably due to relaxation of the joint capsule allowing the femoral head to slide further forward within the acetabulum (Somerville, 1957). The differential diagnosis from other

259

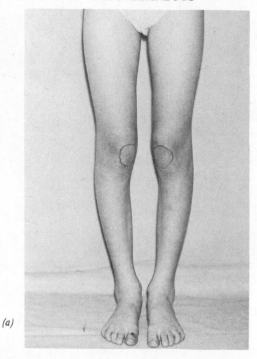

Figure 7.24. Anteversion. (a) The patellae face inwards and the feet forwards due to secondary external torsion of the tibia. (b) The sitting position favoured by children with persistent anteversion

forms of in-toeing, i.e. outward curved tibiae, compensating knock-knees, etc., is usually obvious. Not infrequently, however, internal rotation simulates knock-knee, especially if the running child is observed from behind when the tibiae will inevitably appear to be directed outwards.

D. ROTATIONAL DEFORMITIES OF THE FEMUR

In most there is no functional disability and only a minor cosmetic blemish. Explanation and reassurance suffice. Splinting by Denis Browne's method or twister cables have no influence upon the outcome (Fabry, MacEwan and Shands, 1973). It seems reasonable, however, to discourage sitting with the knees bent and hips flexed in full internal rotation — the television position. A few, however, are handicapped by the deformity, being clumsy, inept at games and in the gymnasium. In some girls the appearance is sufficiently distressing to amount to a disability. Both functional and cosmetic symptoms are aggravated when external rotation of the hips is reduced to less than 20° and compensatory external tibial torsion develops. Furthermore, these opposing rotational malformations are centred upon the knee joint and it is possible that degenerative changes may follow (Guran et al., 1963). The hip may be similarly affected (Somerville, 1957) but as yet there is insufficient evidence for us to recommend surgical correction on these grounds alone (*Figure 7.24*).

The nature of the condition and its relationship to congenital dysplasia of the hip merit consideration. The anteversion angle in the normal baby measures about 40°. This decreases with growth to reach the adult figure of about 12°, the most rapid change occurring within the first 3 years. When this derotation fails, the synonym 'persistent fetal alignment' (Somerville, 1957) becomes apt. The mechanism by which corrective moulding occurs is uncertain, Somerville suggests that pressure of the capsule on the femoral neck in extension is the main factor. It is certainly true that children who habitually sleep with hips in internal rotation are frequently slow to derotate. Walking may also influence resolution for persistent anteversion coupled with coxa valga is commonplace in association with significant delay in the mentally defective (*Figure 7.22*).

In most, however, there is no satisfactory explanation and we must speculate upon the possibility of a primary developmental fault representing in minor degree one aspect of the spectrum of congenital dysplasia. Support is provided by the female prevalence, bilaterality, and a familial trend. Furthermore, it is frequently seen in the opposite hip in unilateral dislocation and in the siblings of children with dislocation. Radiological investigations have localized the fault to the proximal femur and exclude torsion of the femoral shaft (Fabry, MacEwen and Shands, 1973; Harris, 1976). Nevertheless, we do not see any failure of acetabular development, which is so common in patients with known dislocation, in whom anteversion is allowed to persist after satisfactory reduction.

The natural history has been studied by Fabry, MacEwen and Shands (1973) (154 patients) and Harris (1976) (270 patients). Harris has conducted a special clinic for many years at The Hospital for Sick Children, to which these children were referred. 270 patients have been followed to skeletal maturity and no patient has been splinted or exposed to any other form of non-surgical treatment. It was believed at one time that significant derotation commonly occurred after the age of 3 years, but this has been shown to be a false impression for there is little, if any change after this age, and the condition stabilizes without further alleviation at between 8 and 9 years. Fabry and his colleagues concur. This does not imply that many children are handicapped by residual anteversion for in most this is either acceptable or well compensated by postural adaptation or tibial torsion of minor degree.

The only mode of effective treatment is surgical. This may either involve external rotation osteotomy of the femurs at subtrochanteric level to obtain an equal range of inward and outward rotation or, when tibial torsion is significant, femoral external and tibial internal rotation osteotomies in combination. Selection will depend upon a consideration of symptoms and physical signs at about 8 years of age. The disability may be assessed in the gymnasium under the supervision of a physiotherapist, but usually there will be a complaint of clumsiness and poor performance in games and athletics in spite of enthusiasm to excel. Occasionally there is pain in the buttock which is possibly due to muscular fatigue as the child tries to maintain as much lateral rotation as possible. Some girls have a cosmetic blemish which amounts to a disability. These symptoms may arise when lateral rotation is less than 20° and they are usually exacerbated rather than ameliorated when compensatory tibial torsion develops. This is best estimated by palpating the malleoli with the knee flexed to 90° and the tibial tubercle pointing directly forwards.

Femoral rotation osteotomies will resolve the problem in most, providing that secondary tibial deformity is not conspicuous. Should this be so, femoral rotation will make lateral tibial torsion more obvious so that this may also require correction. It is possible that tibial torsion may increase beyond the age of 8 years and consequently operation, once indicated, should not be delayed. Indeed, on occasion, tibial torsion may dominate and then the operation may be confined to the tibia. It is in these patients that we see a most severe form of everted and pronated feet which may be, to some extent, improved if on walking the knees are flexed.

The proportion for whom operation is considered to be warranted will of course vary between surgeons. Harris has operated upon 15 per cent of 270 patients, but some of these were older patients referred to him from elsewhere because of their severity, so that the 15 per cent represents a higher incidence than we would expect in an unselected group. Ten to twelve per cent is probably a close approximation. Of these, two-thirds had femoral osteotomies alone, one-third femoral and tibial osteotomies, and in a very few the operation was confined to the tibia.

The results of operation are satisfying to the patient and parents and it is important to emphasize that the improvement is manifest mainly in performance though the improvement in appearance cannot be ignored. It is a mistake, however, to regard this operation as merely a cosmetic embellishment. This is one of the occasions when pre- and postoperative cinephotography will dispel such misgivings.

(b) Retroversion

When the child first stands, or even earlier, one or both legs are found to be rotated outwards and this is particularly evident in the position of the feet. In essence the clinical features are the opposite of those found in anteversion in that we now find that external rotation of the extended hip is increased at the expense of internal rotation.

Harris (1976) has also reviewed about 120 such patients and has confirmed by radiography that the femoral neck is usually retroverted. In some, however, soft-tissue contracture (involving presumably the short lateral rotators) contributes. This is perhaps not surprising for there is a close correlation with a prone

262

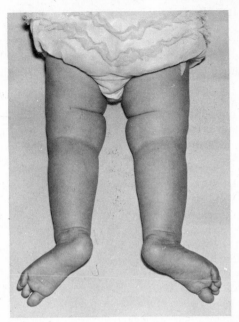

Figure 7.25. Retroversion. (a) The sleeping position

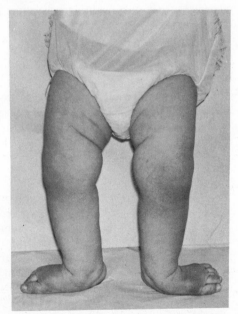

Figure 7.25. (b) The standing position with externally rotated hips and everted feet

sleeping posture in infancy with legs either extended and laterally rotated or in the frog-leg position, both of which will favour both the skeletal and muscular elements (Harris, 1972). Sometimes only one leg is held in this position and then the deformity may be unilateral (*Figure 7.25*).

The outcome is quite different from that seen when anteversion is present. Very few persist beyond the age of 3 years (with the exception of some of negro descent), and of those that do we have yet to see one for whom operation seemed justified or even likely to be necessary in the future. We may reasonably assume that as the prone sleeping position becomes less consistent with increasing age, so the deforming pressure on the femoral neck decreases and contracted muscles are subjected to correcting forces. This, however, is not the whole explanation for some do not sleep in this position and they cannot be so explained. The prognosis is, nevertheless, equally good and compensatory tibial torsion does not develop.

E. BONE TUMOURS AND CYSTS

A catalogue of remote possibilities will serve no purpose, for many of the neoplasms, benign and malignant, which are of diagnostic significance in the adult are by their rarity of little practical importance in this age group, e.g. osteoclastoma and plasmocytoma. Similarly there are lesions which, although occurring in children, seldom if ever affect the hip joint, e.g. osteoclastoma, chondroblastoma and fibrous cortical defect. There remain those which both affect children and which are found in and around the hip joint. Detailed descriptions of the macro- and microscopic features may, if desired, be obtained elsewhere; only those aspects of clinical and therapeutic significance will be mentioned below.

1. Benign lesions

These include osteochondroma, osteoid osteoma, aneurysmal bone cyst, localized eosinophilic granuloma, simple solitary cysts and localized fibrous dysplasia, and lastly, subacute or chronic infective conditions.

Osteoid osteoma

This has a predilection for the trochanteric area and this area is the commonest site in children. The clinical features of an aching pain which gets worse at night and which is relieved by salicylates are common to all sites but when the tumour is near a joint the signs may suggest that the joint is primarily at fault. Thus, the hip may be irritable resembling an arthritis with muscle-wasting and the radiograph may disclose widespread regional osteoporosis. In the past, confusion has arisen with tuberculous arthritis, especially when the tumour is translucent rather than sclerotic (Spence and Lloyd-Roberts, 1961). Even if suspected, it may be difficult to identify on routine radiographs when reactive sclerosis either obscures the nidus and suggests infection, or, being in the translucent form, it introduces uncertainty in differentiation from a bone island. Oblique projections, tomography and bone-scanning may be aids to diagnosis. Although the symptoms will disappear in between 2 and 6 years (Golding, 1954), removal is obviously desirable and excision must include the whole tumour or recurrence is probable.

E. BONE TUMOURS AND CYSTS

This may be particularly difficult in an extensive area of cancellous bone such as we find in the trochanteric region. Block excision under radiographic control and identification of the red or grey nidus encased in dense bone is the method most likely to succeed.

Aneurysmal bone cyst

In children this has certain properties which distinguish it from the adult pattern. It is usually situated in the metaphyseal area of a long bone (*Figure 7.26*) or in the vertebral adnexa where it expands rapidly and is well described as resembling

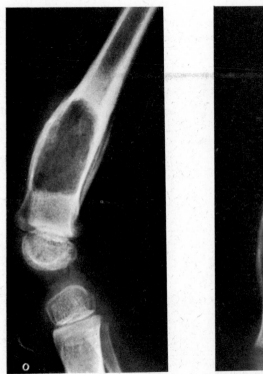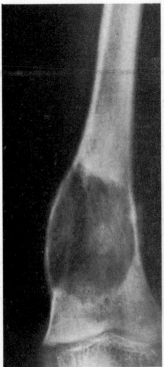

Figure 7.26. Aneurysmal bone cyst. The characteristic appearance in young children

bubble gum. This capacity for rapid expansion with penetration of the growth plate and invasion of the epiphysis is, in a long bone, associated with pain, local tenderness and stretching, reddening, and venous engorgement of the overlying skin. The resemblance to a malignant tumour is obvious and at operation the appearance may be equally misleading for the cavity is full of blood and the expanded walls are little more than thickened fibrous tissue with a thin lining of bone. In such vigorous lesions excision, bone-grafting, and arthrodesis of the nearby joint is the only possibility and even amputation may be necessary in more aggressive examples. In those less aggressive curettage with bone-grafting followed by radiotherapy, especially in inaccessible areas, may be followed by healing. In one patient with femoral involvement, destruction was so extensive that excision and repair were not possible, amputation was performed and histological confirmation of the diagnosis obtained. The patient died later with pulmonary metastases so it would seem that in some tumours there is a frontier between the benign aneurysmal bone cyst and a malignant angiosarcoma.

Localized eosinophilic granuloma

Although the trochanteric area may be involved in generalized histiocytosis (Hand-Schueller-Christian) by an expanding and destructive cyst causing coxa vara or a pathological fracture, the localized variety tends to be clearly demarcated

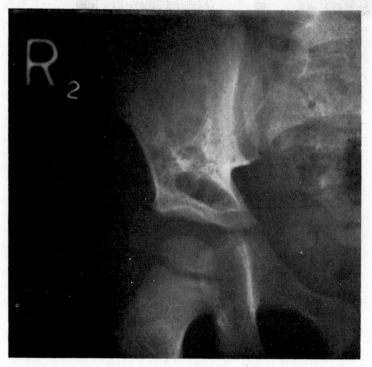

Figure 7.27. Eosinophilic granuloma within the roof of the acetabulum.
(Reproduced from Lloyd-Roberts, *Orthopaedics in Infancy and Childhood,* 1971, Butterworths, by permission)

and less prone to these complications. The trochanteric lesion is trabeculated, somewhat expanded and surrounded by a sclerotic margin, unlike those in the diaphysis which stimulate periosteal reaction of the onion-peel variety. Local lesions tend to heal spontaneously so it is difficult to assess the contribution of radiotherapy, curettage and grafting though this may be indicated if there is anxiety about stability. Oblique and lateral radiographs may be helpful in showing a surprising amount of uninvolved normal bone. The pelvis is also a favourite site. The lesion is enclosed within the ilium, being either discrete above the acetabular roof (*Figure 7.27*), or diffuse within the wing. In spite of the apparently perilous position of acetabular granulomata, they seem to heal without affecting the hip joint.

Simple cysts and localized fibrous dysplasia

These may be considered together for they have both similarities and differences. They may be indistinguishable on radiological examination but fibrous dysplasia is the more likely in this situation. Both are prone to fracture, are followed by union with deformity and have no great tendency to heal as a result of this. Spontaneous healing is more likely to occur in simple cysts and curettage and grafting are more likely to succeed, especially when the cysts are separated from the growth plate by normal bone. Furthermore, cysts move in their entirety away from the plate as growth proceeds, but fibrous dysplasia remains stationary with a tendency to expand distally. At operation, cysts are filled with serous fluid, are lined by a thin membrane, and are unilocular with ridges on the walls; fibrous dysplasia is multilocular, and filled with grey, gritty, fibrous tissue. The localized form of fibrous dysplasia is more common than the polyostotic variety and has a greater tendency to spontaneous healing. Both varieties are seen predominantly in the proximal femur.

Treatment of the two is similar. If the lesions are large enough to hazard stability or are painful (indicating a crack fracture), operation is indicated. Curettage and cancellous bone-grafting with nail-plate fixation is the method of choice, but sometimes a specially made long plate will be necessary if fibrous dysplasia has expanded distally into the shaft (*Figure 7.7*). Before operation the surgeon may doubt the potential security of fixation of the nail component, but in practice there is enough normal bone remaining to ensure this. As already mentioned, we may expect simple cysts to heal by this method, but this is far less likely in fibrous dysplasia in which coxa vara is prone to progress. The operation must then be repeated, together with abduction osteotomy. Grafts have a tendency to be absorbed and often the size of the cavity will strain our resources of autogenous bone. It is then better to concentrate our reinforcement to the area of the calcar femorale (Garceau and Gregory, 1954; Henry, 1969).

Cysts in subacute and chronic osteomyelitis

The thick-walled chronic metaphyseal abscess with central sequestrum is unlikely to be misinterpreted but the subacute cystic form may well be. This is seen as a cyst with ill-defined edges or a thin cortical margin which may expand to cross the growth plate. Coxa magna, reflecting local hyperaemia, is common. Clinically there is pain, tenderness, marked muscle-wasting, and sometimes limitation of hip movement. It is usually necessary to confirm the diagnosis by biopsy and culture but the response to the appropriate antibiotic is usually satisfactory (Harris and Kirkaldy-Willis, 1965).

2. Malignant tumours

Primary tumours

These include *Osteogenic sarcoma, Chondrosarcoma* and *Ewing's tumour* but their incidence is low in children under 12 years. Osteogenic sarcoma for example, is a condition which arises predominantly between the ages of 10 and 25 years but of these no more than 4 per cent present in children under 12, of which most occur in situations other than the hip, notably the knee and humerus. Indeed we have seen but 1 and that arose in the femoral neck within the exuberant callus of a fracture in a child with osteogenesis imperfecta (Klenerman, Ockenden and Townsend, 1967). Similarly chondrosarcoma, whether arising *de novo* or superimposed upon a pre-existing chondroma, is more likely to be seen in adult life but shows at all ages a predilection for the pelvis. Ewing's tumour, rare though it is, arises predominantly under the age of 20 years, may affect young children and favours the pelvic bones, especially the ilium.

The recent development of effective chemotherapy has thrown our pre-conceived notions of prognosis and management into confusion. This impact is seen most dramatically when the pulmonary metastases of osteogenic sarcoma are seen to fade away whether they be large cannon-balls or seedlings demonstrable only on tomography. While awaiting the outcome of prospective clinical trials (in this country that organized by the Medical Research Council seems to be showing promising results in favour of chemotherapy) we must clearly adapt our management to these new developments. When feasible, primary amputation is followed by irradiation of the lungs and high doses of methotrexate continued, it would seem, for at least a year. We may with some optimism hope to see an improvement upon the 12 to 15 per cent 5-year survival rate generally achieved before the introduction of chemotherapy.

Unfortunately, however, the same optimism cannot be extended to chondrosarcoma and Ewing's tumour. Chondrosarcomas are both radioresistant and respond poorly to chemotherapy, so that surgical excision remains the only effective method of treatment. Similarly Ewing's tumour, although radio-sensitive and affected by chemotherapeutic drugs, has a tendency to escape from these restraining influences in time. At the moment a local sterilizing dose of radiation, which aims to reach a level of 6 000 Rads, followed by actinomycin or cyclophosphamide is the favoured mode of treatment. Unfortunately however, respect for pelvic viscera will reduce the optimum dose of irradiation for pelvic tumours to a less desirable level.

Secondary tumours

These tumours, if not metastases of primary bone tumours elsewhere or retinoblastoma, arise for practical purposes from neuroblastoma. The pelvis is a common site for these metastases but unfortunately once these are seen the outcome is almost invariably fatal. Spontaneous maturation to ganglioneuroma or successful excision of a primary tumour presenting as an abdominal mass arising from the suprarenal medulla or seen on the chest radiograph when the site of origin is a sympathetic ganglion, seldom affect the outcome. If the primary tumour is not apparent, diagnosis may be difficult for the histological distinction between neuroblastoma and Ewing's tumour may be finely drawn. Similarly, the radiological features may closely resemble one another.

We should remember, however, that neuroblastoma is a tumour of early life occurring commonly within the first year and it may even be present at birth, whereas Ewing's tumour tends to present later. Identification of the catecholamine derivative, vanillylmandelic acid (V.M.A.), in the urine will, however, confirm neuroblastoma in some 60 per cent of patients. Orthopaedic treatment of pathological fractures around the hip is inevitably no more than symptomatic but radiotherapy may relieve pain and chemotherapy provide some temporary palliation.

F. DISORDERS OF THE HAEMOPOIETIC SYSTEM

Haemophilia

Haemophilia and allied coagulation defects may affect the hip and its surroundings. Arthropathy rarely involves the hip joint itself, in contrast to the knee and elbow, but metaphyseal haemorrhagic cysts may develop (*Figure 7.28*) and haemorrhage into surrounding muscles may cause deformity indirectly. Should, however,

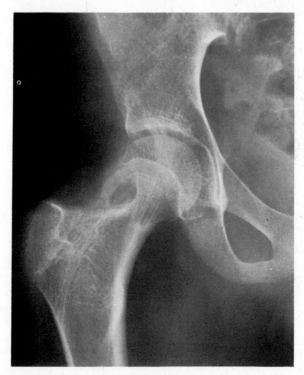

Figure 7.28. A haemophiliac bone cyst is present in the neck of the femur but the joint is unaffected

269

recurrent episodes involve the joint, secondary ischaemic necrosis of the capital epiphyses is a probable complication which will contribute to disorganization predisposing to further haemorrhage. Intramuscular haemorrhage is liable to affect the iliacus when, as a result of developing tension within its sheath, the femoral nerve may be affected. The pseudotumours which occur in the buttock and thigh are at first encysted haematomas which gradually enlarge to threaten major vessels and nerves and finally the skin. Excision may be taxing but must be complete, for incision is followed by further bleeding and the risk of secondary infection. Fractures are probably best treated by internal fixation to reduce the area of exposed bleeding bone and to overcome the problem of severe unsuspected haemorrhage occurring within a plaster.

These are the complications which we recognized in the past and treated by a combination of rest, traction, splinting and, on occasion, by surgery, providing that the deficient coagulation Factor VIII could be raised sufficiently by the substitution measures available at the time. Now, however, human antihaemophilic globulin prepared as cryoprecipitate is being produced in sufficient quantity for both hospital and domiciliary use. This development seems likely to revolutionize management for, if cryoprecipitate is used, as soon as there is evidence of spontaneous or traumatic haemorrhage, control is effective. We may reasonably hope that the classical complications will be prevented in the future and that if they do arise they may be treated by established conservative and surgical methods without risk to the patient.

Sickle cell anaemia

This is seen with increasing frequency because of our new immigrant population from the West Indies. There is also an affected community in the eastern Mediterranean, notably northern Greece, where it is not infrequently seen in company with thalassaemia. Thalassaemia does not affect joints except as a component of marrow hyperplasia which may cause coxa magna. Anaemia and its complications are found almost exclusively in those with the homozygous SS variety but we have learnt recently that bone changes may also appear very rarely when the trait (haemoglobin S) is present. The hip joint is not surprisingly a frequent target for the bone changes are the result of intra-osseous thrombosis to which the circulation of the femoral head is particularly vulnerable.

The appearances resemble those of Perthes' disease, and may be unilateral or bilateral and necrosis segmental or complete. The infarcts are not confined to childhood and may present in middle-age when the haematological defect is more likely to be of the SC or S-Thalassaemia varieties. This may be because SS disease is often fatal before bone changes become evident. Pain varies from severe to negligible and may be overshadowed by pain in the abdomen. The influence of low oxygen tension in pathogenesis is well known and its cause may have been congestive heart failure, pneumonia or anaesthesia administered without due precaution. Unlike sickle cell bone infarcts elsewhere, there is no special tendency to secondary infection.

The outcome is related to age at onset and the proportion of the head involved. Thus in the young with segmental necrosis the outcome is likely to be favourable in terms of head shape and symptoms, whereas an adult with total necrosis is not

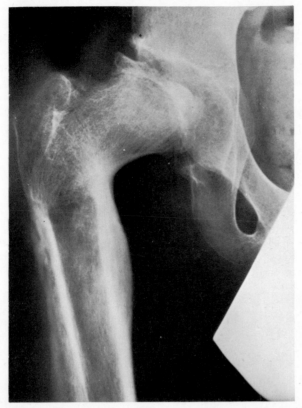

Figure 7.29. Sickle cell anaemia. Severe residual deformity of the femoral head in spite of varus rotation osteotomy. The nail plate has been removed

so favoured. The similarity to Perthes' disease in the young inevitably stimulates speculation about containment treatment for those in whom it would seem indicated in Perthes' disease. We must await the results from centres treating numbers of these patients and in the meantime rely on methods which protect the hip from weight-bearing during the painful stage (Chung and Ralston, 1969) (*Figure 7.29*).

Leukaemia

This may declare itself to the orthopaedic surgeon in the first instance and the symptoms may arise in the pelvic area. A somewhat pasty child with vague aching pains in the limbs or referred pain from the spine may give a history of recurrent infection and undue bruising. The radiograph discloses osteoporosis with small areas of translucent erosion and sometimes unexplained periostitis. Larger osteolytic tumour-like areas and pathological fractures are unusual but lines of metaphyseal translucency and multiple vertebral collapse are not uncommon. The overall clinical picture may be confused with juvenile rheumatoid arthritis. In children acute lymphoblastic leukaemia accounts for 80 per cent but primitive blast cells may not always be identifiable in peripheral blood in the early stages or during remissions. Hypochromic anaemia, thrombocytopenia and a raised sedimentation rate are diagnostic indicators. Examination of the bone marrow is essential. Therapeutic advances have overtaken our ability to forecast the outcome. Contrived remission with prednisone and vincristine, followed by cranial irradiation and intrathecal methotrexate, maintains remission in about 50 per cent of patients for 3 years and it is hoped that some 30 per cent who are in long-term remission may be cured. Unfortunately there is no evidence that prompt diagnosis has a favourable influence on the outcome.

G. METABOLIC DISEASES

Rickets characterized by osteoporosis, coxa vara, pelvic deformity and meta-physeal translucency is a feature of a variety of childhood diseases of which some may be referred to orthopaedic surgeons in the first instance. Among these are the nutritional (*Figure 7.30*) and Vitamin-D resistant (*Figure 7.31*)

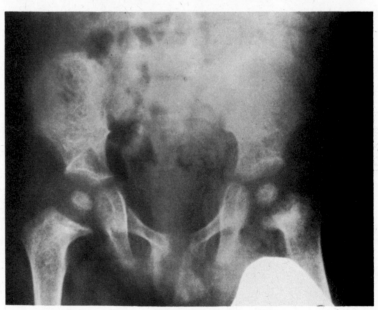

Figure 7.30. Nutritional rickets. Unusually florid changes at the hips

varieties for whom the prognosis is greatly improved if diagnosis is prompt. Others are more likely to present first to paediatricians as undefined sick children who later or incidently show evidence of rickets. Renal and hepatic failure, cystinosis and Wilson's disease are examples (*Figure 7.32*). Malabsorption syndromes occur in children and the so-called idiopathic osteoporosis of ado-lescence may be a reflection of this disorder.

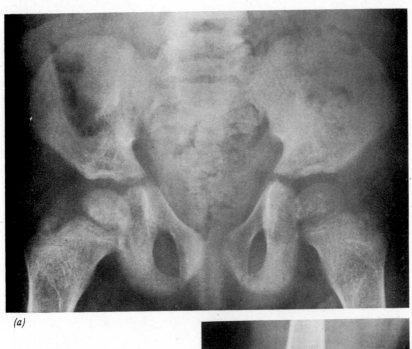

(a)

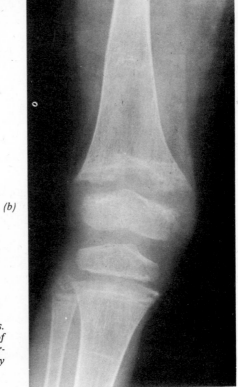

(b)

*Figure 7.31. Vitamin-D resistant rickets.
(a) In the pelvis the appearances are of
osteoporosis. (b) The changes characteristic of rickets tend to be seen at rapidly
growing epiphyseal plates*

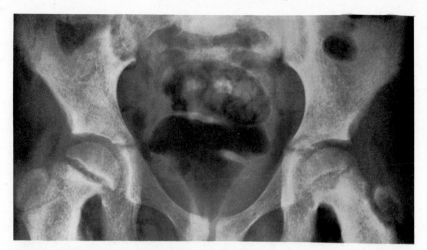

Figure 7.32. Renal rickets. Note widening of the growth plate causing some epiphyseal displacement on the right. There is some erosion of the calcar and the trabecular pattern is exaggerated

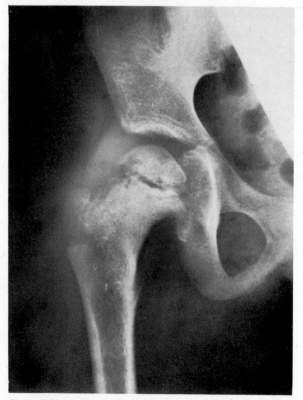

Figure 7.33. Gaucher's disease. (a) There are areas of infiltration in the metaphysis and head. The hip was irritable

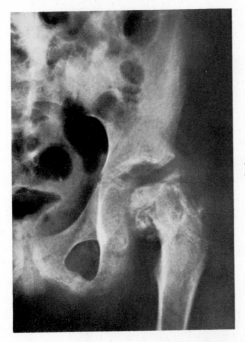

Figure 7.33. (b) Six months later the head has collapsed. There was severe pain

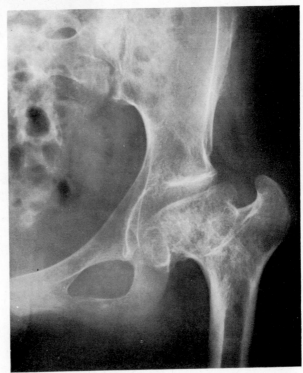

Figure 7.33. (c) Ten years later. Restricted movement but no pain

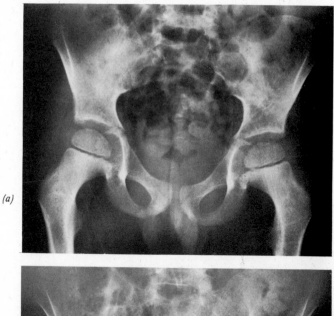

(a)

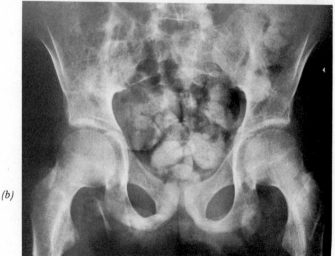

(b)

Figure 7.34. The hips in homocystinuria. (a) At 7 years of age the femoral shafts and necks are thin, the metaphyses flared and there is coxa magna. (b) Four years later at 11 years these changes are established

The *Mucopolysaccharidoses* are identifiable by an increase in urinary excretion of this substance. The hips are involved in all the clinical subgroups which include Gargoylism, Morquio, Sanfilippo and Maroteaux-Lamy.

In *Gaucher's disease* the bones are infiltrated by Kerasin — a lipoid cerebroside. The femoral epiphysis may be affected and there is a resemblance to Perthes' disease in the early stages followed later by collapse and deformity (*Figure 7.33*). Pain may be severe at first but abates with time. Relief of pain is difficult but success has been seen to follow both irradiation and epiphyseal curettage.

In *Homocystinuria* there is porosis with coxa magna (*Figure 7.34*) and rarely Perthes-simulating changes. Similarly in *Hypercalcaemia* due to hypervitaminosis D we may see increased density of the femoral epiphysis.

H. OSTEOCHONDRITIS DISSECANS

Osteochondritis dissecans of the femoral head in childhood is very rare. Guilleminet and Barbier (1957) described the clinical details of 8 cases but only 2 were children, one a boy aged 12 years and the other a girl aged 11 years; both presented with pain. The radiographical appearance is of a translucency in the superior portion of the femoral head with a central avascular fragment. In contrast to osteochondritis dissecans, at other sites loose bodies do not occur.

In recent years, interest has been particularly shown in the occurrence of this condition following Legge–Calvé–Perthes disease (Hallel and Salvati, 1976; Kamhi and MacEwen, 1975; and Ratliff, 1967). Only 2 of the total 51 cases in the literature were treated surgically (Kamhi and MacEwen, 1975). Hallel and Salvati (1976) described the histology of two young adults who had surgical treatment with relief of symptoms. In both there were dead bony trabeculae surrounded by living fibrocartilage. These findings tend to support the suggestion of Ratliff that an unhealed necrotic bone fragment may persist from the time of active disease into adult life. Ratliff (1967) reported 2 patients followed for 30 years without healing but with good hips. One of these has now been followed for 42 years (Ratliff, 1967; case I) (*Figure 7.35 (a) (b)* and *(c)*). Thus it would appear that surgical treatment is very rarely required.

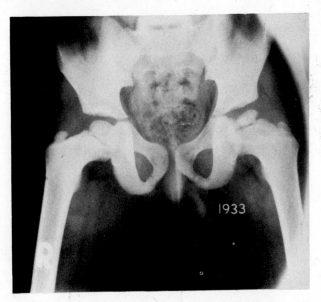

Figure 7.35. (a) Radiograph of a hip in 1933 at the age of 7 years. There is flattening of the upper femoral epiphysis and an area of increased density in the centre of the epiphysis

277

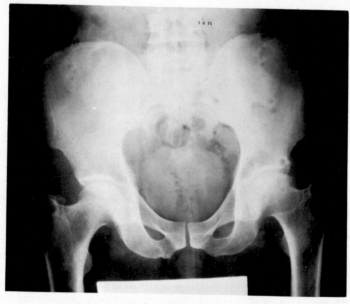

(b)

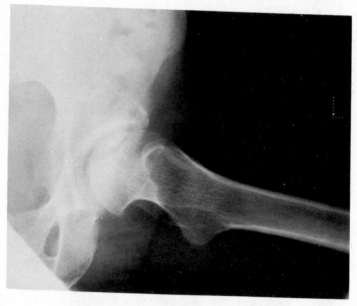

(c)

Figure 7.35. (b), (c). Radiographs in 1975 when aged 49. There were no symptoms and full movements in the left hip. Minor cystic changes have developed in the lateral part of the acetabulum in the last 10 years

I. TRANSIENT SYNOVITIS

This condition has been variously called the observation hip, the irritable hip and coxalgia (a fleeting pain in the hip). It is generally conceded to be the commonest cause of a painful hip in childhood (Wiles, 1951; Ferguson, 1954).

Clinical features

The clinical picture is well recognized (Adams, 1963; de Valderrama, 1963; Hardinge, 1970).

Transient synovitis mainly affects children under the age of 10 years and it occurs more commonly in boys than in girls. The onset may be abrupt or insidious. Symptoms vary in severity. They may be fleeting and last for a few days but more rarely for several weeks. The pain in the hip may radiate to the thigh or knee. Signs are variable. There may be mild restriction of movement or acute spasm with severe restriction of all movement. Local tenderness is usually only slight. The clinical presentation is similar to that of Perthes' disease but the radiographs are normal. An increase in joint space with capsular thickening has been described but it is seldom impressive.

Characteristically, the patient has a normal or slightly raised temperature and erythrocyte sedimentation rate and a normal white blood count. In no case reported in the literature has any bacteria ever been isolated from joint biopsy or aspiration (Hardinge, 1970). The symptoms usually rapidly subside with a few days' rest in bed, though in a small number of patients more prolonged immobilization has been required (de Valderrama, 1963).

Aetiology

This has been the subject of considerable investigation but remains unknown; Miller (1931) and Butler (1933) suggested a low grade bone or joint infection but this has never been proved. Blockey and Porter (1968) reported negative results from a methodical search for evidence of a viral infection. They concluded that trauma probably remains the most frequent explanation but this is obviously difficult to prove or disprove in a young child. Hardinge (1970) performed a careful prospective study on 65 patients. He found no connection with infection, either bacterial or viral, allergy or trauma.

Transient synovitis affects a similar age group to Perthes' disease and it is natural that a causal relationship should be suspected. This may be supported by the work of Kemp (1973) since he induced Perthes'-like changes in small dogs by producing an artificial effusion in the hip joint. However, the evidence is inconclusive at the present time. Spock (1959) reviewed the literature and found an incidence of Perthes' disease in children who had previously suffered from transient synovitis of only 1.5 per cent, while Adams (1963) found no cases at all in a follow-up on 50 children.

Perthes' disease developing several months after an episode of transient synovitis is well recognized and observation should be continued for several months with radiographs, but the association is rare.

Diagnosis and treatment

The child with an irritable hip should be investigated at once to exclude more serious disease. In the majority of cases with a normal radiograph, temperature, and erythrocyte sedimentation rate, there is no debate on diagnosis. If the child is ill then the possibility of tuberculosis, suppurative arthritis, osteomyelitis of the neck of the femur, and early rheumatoid arthritis must be remembered. If there is any doubt concerning diagnosis, then bed-rest with gentle traction in hospital for a short period of about a week is necessary. All these conditions are excluded either by investigations or by the subsequent course of the disease. Alternatively, the child may rest at home in bed.

Prognosis

Complete recovery is usually expected. However, de Valderrama (1963) examined the possible sequelae of this disorder by studying 23 patients, 15 to 30 years later. Varying degrees of coxa magna, osteoarthritis, or simple broadening of the femoral neck were found in 12 of the 23 patients studied. Valderrama considered that the changes may be a 'consequence of hypervascularization of the bone'. Though the author has seen several patients with radiological abnormalities some years after transient synovitis of the hip, none have required treatment.

REFERENCES

Adams, J. A. (1963). Transient synovitis of the hip joint in children. *J. Bone Jt Surg.* **45B**, 471

Axer, A. (1958). Transposition of gluteus maximus, tensor fasciae latae and iliotibial band for paralysis of lateral abdominal muscles in children after poliomyelitis. A preliminary report. *J. Bone Jt Surg.* **40B**, 644

Beighton, P. and Horan, F. (1969). Orthopaedic aspects of the Ehlers-Danlos syndrome. *J. Bone Jt Surg.* **51B**, 444

Blockey, N. J. and Porter, B. B. (1968). Transient synovitis of the hip: a virological investigation. *Br. Med. J.* **4**, 557

Brenton, D. P., Dow, C. J., James, J. I. P., Hay, R. L., and Wynne-Davies, R. (1972). Homocystinuria and Marfan's Syndrome. A comparison. *J. Bone Jt Surg.* **54B**, 277

Butler, R. W. (1933). Transitory arthritis of the hip joint in childhood. *Br. Med. J.* **1**, 951

Carroll, N. G. and Sharrard, W. J. W. (1972). Long-term follow-up of posterior iliopsoas transplantation for paralytic dislocation of the hip. *J. Bone Jt Surg.* **54A**, 551

Carter, C., and Wilkinson, J. (1964). Persistent joint laxity and congenital dislocation of the hip. *J. Bone Jt Surg.* **46B**, 40

Chung, S. M. K. and Ralston, E. L. (1969). Necrosis of the femoral head associated with sickle-cell anemia and its genetic variants. *J. Bone Jt Surg.* **51A**, 33

Fabry, G., MacEwen, G. D. and Shands, A. R. (1973). Torsion of the femur. A follow-up study in normal and abnormal conditions. *J. Bone Jt Surg.* **55A**, 1726

Ferguson, A. B. (1954). Synovitis of the hip and Legg–Perthes disease. *Clin. Orthop.* **4**, 180

Garceau, G. J. and Gregory, C. F. (1954). Solitary unicameral bone cyst. *J. Bone Jt Surg.* **36A**, 267

Golding, J. S. R. (1954). The natural history of osteoid osteoma. *J. Bone Jt Surg.* **36B**, 218

REFERENCES

Guilleminet, M. and Barbier, J. M. (1957). Osteochondritis dissecans of the hip. *J. Bone Jt Surg.* **39B**, 268

Gunn, D. R. (1964). Contracture of the quadriceps muscle. A discussion on the aetiology and relationship to recurrent dislocation of the patella. *J. Bone Jt Surg.* **46B**, 492

Guran, P., Masse, P., Bruchon, D. and Salet, J. (1963). Conséquences cliniques de l'antéversion exagérée ducol fémoral (en l'absence de toute autre malformation associée). *Archs fr. Pédiat.* **20**, 856

Hallel, T. and Salvati, E. A. (1976). Osteochondritis dissecans following Legg–Calvé–Perthes disease. *J. Bone Jt Surg.* **58A**, 708

Hardinge, K. (1970). The etiology of transient synovitis of the hip in childhood. *J. Bone Jt Surg.* **52B**, 100

Harris, N. H. (1961). Myositis ossificans progressiva. *Proc. R. Soc. Med.* **54**, 70

Harris, N. H. and Kirkaldy-Willis, W. H. (1965). Primary subacute pyogenic osteomyelitis. *J. Bone Jt Surg.* **47B**, 526

Harris, N. H. (1972). Rotational deformities and their secondary effects in the lower extremities in children. *J. Bone Jt Surg.* **54B**, 172

Harris, N. H. (1976). Personal communication

Henry, A. (1969). Monostotic fibrous dysplasia *J. Bone Jt Surg.* **51B**, 300

Kamhi, E. and MacEwen, G. D. (1975). Osteochondritis dissecans in Legg–Calvé–Perthes disease. *J. Bone Jt Surg.* **75A**, 506

Kemp, H. B. S. (1973). Perthes' disease: an experimental and clinical study. *Ann. R. Coll. Surg.* **52**, 18

Klenerman, L., Ockenden, B. G. and Townsend, A. C. (1967). Osteosarcoma occurring in osteogenesis imperfecta. *J. Bone Jt Surg.* **49B**, 314

Laurence, K. M. (1964). The natural history of spina bifida cystica. *Archs Dis. Childh.* **39**, 41

Lloyd-Roberts, G. C. and Lettin, A. W. F. (1970). Arthrogryposis multiplex congenita. *J. Bone Jt Surg.* **52B**, 494

Lloyd-Roberts, G. C. and Thomas, T. G. (1964). The aetiology of quadriceps contracture in children. *J. Bone Jt Surg.* **46B**, 498

Menelaus, M. B. (1971). *The Orthopaedic Management of Spina Bifida Cystica.* Edinburgh: Livingstone

Miller, O. L. (1931). Acute transient epiphysitis of the hip joint. *J. Am. Med. Ass.* **96**, 575

Mustard, W. T. (1959). A follow-up study of iliopsoas transfer for hip instability. *J. Bone Jt Surg.* **41B**, 289

Parsons, D. W. and Seddon, H. J. (1968). The results of operations for disorders of the hip caused by poliomyelitis. *J. Bone Jt Surg.* **50B**, 266

Ratliff, A. H. C. (1967). Osteochondritis dissecans following Legg–Calvé–Perthes disease. *J. Bone Jt Surg.* **49B**, 108

Rubin, P. (1964). *Dynamic Classification of Bone Dysplasias.* Chicago: Yearbook Medical Publishers Inc.

Samilson, R. L., Tsou, P., Aamoth, G. and Green, W. M. (1972). Dislocation and subluxation of the hip in cerebral palsy: pathogenesis, natural history, and management. *J. Bone Jt Surg.* **54A**, 863

Seymour, N. and Sharrard, W. J. W. (1968). Bilateral proximal release of the hamstrings in cerebral palsy. *J. Bone Jt Surg.* **50B**, 274

Sharrard, W. J. W. (1964). Posterior iliopsoas transplantation in the treatment of paralytic dislocation of the hip. *J. Bone Jt Surg.* **46B**, 426

Sharrard, W. J. W. (1971). *Paediatric Orthopaedics and Fractures.* Oxford: Blackwell Scientific Publications

Somerville, E. W. (1957). Persistent foetal alignment of the hip. *J. Bone Jt Surg.* **39B**, 106

Spence, A. J. and Lloyd-Roberts, G. C. (1961). Regional osteoporosis in osteoid osteoma. *J. Bone Jt Surg.* **43B**, 501

Spock, A. (1959). Transient synovitis of the hip joint in children. *Paediatrics,* **24**, 1042

Spranger, J. W., Langer, L. O. and Wiedemann, H. R. (1974). *Bone Dysplasias. An Atlas of Constitutional Disorders of Skeletal Development.* Philadelphia: W. B. Saunders Co.

Stephenson, C. T. and Donovan, M. M. (1969). Transfer of hip adductor origins to the ischium in spastic cerebral palsy. *J. Bone Jt Surg.* **51A**, 1040

REFERENCES

Valderrama, J. A. F. de (1963). The observation hip syndrome and its late sequelae. *J. Bone Jt Surg.* **45B,** 462

Wiles, P. (1951). *Essentials of Orthopaedics,* p. 134. London: J. & A. Churchill

Wynne-Davies, R. and Fairbank, T. J. (1976). *Fairbank's Atlas of General Affections of the Skeleton.* Edinburgh: Churchill Livingstone

Index